INSOMNIA DECODED

BREAK THE CYCLE OF SLEEPLESS NIGHTS

AUDREY PORTER

CONTENTS

INTRODUCTION

> *People say, "I'm going to sleep now," as if it were noth-ing. But it's really a bizarre activity. "For the next several hours, while the sun is gone, I'm going to become unconscious, temporarily losing command over every-thing I know and understand. When the sun returns, I will resume my life."*

— GEORGE CARLIN

It's yet another fruitless night of tossing and turning. Another hour of staring at the ceiling in the dark. Another instance of doing the math to see how many hours of sleep you will get if you fall asleep *right now*. Another night of convincing yourself to *please go to sleep*.

Welcome to *Decoding Insomnia*. Here, we will address the typical challenges you face with sleep and delve into potential solutions. In this book, we'll look at the science of sleep, what insomnia is, and how to know if you have it. Then, we'll look at a few different ways you can manage it and get better quality rest.

A little about me, first: I am a physician. Many of my patients have sleep disorders like insomnia. This book aims to equip patients with the knowledge and tools they need to succeed.

Statistics show that roughly 70 million Americans have some sleep disorder. Nearly 30% of all adults will experience a form of insomnia during their lifetime, making it the most common sleep disorder. Of these people, a third will develop long-term or chronic insomnia.

I'm sure you understand the significant negative impact of insomnia on your overall quality of life. No one likes not getting enough sleep, and there are few things quite as frustrating as waking up feeling more tired than when you went to bed. Sleep is essential to our well-being. The constant struggle to fall asleep and stay asleep can have a lasting impact on both your physical and mental health.

Recent statistics show that roughly 40% of insomniacs have diagnosable mental health conditions such as depression, social anxiety disorder (SAD), and post-traumatic stress disorder (PTSD). A staggering 83% of people with depression experience insomnia symptoms, while 91% of people with PTSD report the same.

Not only is it prevalent, but insomnia can also have life-altering consequences. If left alone, insomnia can lead to

- fatigue
- mood changes
- sleep deprivation
- reduced judgment, worsening cognitive abilities, and weaker overall performance at work or school
- increased risks while driving or walking
- higher chance of developing cardiovascular issues (like high blood pressure), asthma, diabetes, and obesity

Luckily, insomnia is manageable. It **does not** have to control your life. There are steps you can take and changes you can make to get better rest.

Now, this book is not intended to supplement proper medical care. You should always consult a doctor before making drastic changes to your lifestyle. While sleep disorders aren't usually symptoms of other issues, they can be—and should be—checked out to ensure that there isn't an underlying health condition. On top of that, certain sleep disorders can be dangerous if not appropriately treated and require medical intervention. If you haven't seen a doctor about your sleep troubles, please consider doing so.

Finally, most of the methods and strategies we discuss in this book take time to fix. They take time and dedication. If something doesn't immediately give you results, give it some time. In the same breath, maintain an open mind. We often write options off as something that won't work before we truly consider them. If you find yourself thinking, "Oh, this won't work for me," take a moment to figure out why you believe that. If you can't find any specific reason, try it.

With all that said, let's begin!

1

UNDERSTANDING WHAT KEEPS YOU UP AT NIGHT

 Am I sleeping? Have I slept at all? This is insomnia.

— CHUCK PALAHNIUK

THE IMPORTANCE OF SLEEP

Let me start by stating that sleep is vital to your body's regulation and dramatically affects your health and well-being. It's often considered as important as a well-balanced diet and regular exercise. Think of it as a kind of scheduled maintenance. Without it, your mind and body would deteriorate a lot faster than they should.

Sleep affects the following areas:

- **Hormones:** Our bodies produce different hormones at different times of the day. For some, production depends on sleep. Growth hormones are increased during sleep, while others are regulated by our sleeping patterns. For example, cortisol is released in the mornings to wake us up and make us more alert. At night, cortisol production is slowed down, and melatonin is produced to make us feel sleepy.
- **Cognitive abilities:** The brain plasticity theory explores why we sleep. It holds that our brains undergo restructuring while we rest. The brain uses the downtime that comes with sleeping to create new neural connections and update existing pathways. This explains why studies have found that good-quality sleep leads to better memory, concentration, problem-solving, and decision-making.
- **Mood and emotional regulation:** How well you sleep influences how well you regulate your emotions. It also affects your overall mood and how likely you are to socialize with others. People who don't get enough rest are less capable of controlling their emotions and less responsive to empathy or humor. This, combined with low energy levels, creates an overall less pleasant disposition.
- **Cardiovascular health:** While you sleep, your heart rate slows, and your blood pressure drops. This gives your cardiovascular system some downtime. Lack of

sleep increases how long these systems stay awake, increasing your risk of cardiovascular complications.

- **Immune system:** During sleep, the body produces cytokines (small proteins released by cells to influence the functioning of other cells). Cytokines work with white blood cells to fight infections. Not getting enough sleep can result in less cytokine production, ultimately leading to a weaker immune system and more frequent infections. On the other hand, better quality sleep leads to optimized cytokine production and a more efficient immune system.

- **Athletic performance:** Growth hormones are at their highest during sleep. These hormones contribute to muscle growth and tissue repair. Getting a good amount of sleep optimizes how well your body can restore muscle damage and thus improves your overall performance.

- **Weight:** You might be surprised that sleep influences weight gain and loss. Sleep impacts the production of two hormones: leptin (an appetite suppressor) and ghrelin (an appetite aggravator). While you sleep, leptin production is increased while ghrelin is decreased. If you do not get enough sleep, the body produces more ghrelin and less leptin, which makes you feel hungry more often and decreases how quickly you feel full. This results in overeating. On top of this, inadequate sleep affects impulse control and stress, which further impact how likely you are to overeat.

How Much Sleep Do You Need?

The ideal amount of sleep per night depends on a few things. The most significant influence is how old you are, and there are scientifically-backed recommendations for how long you should sleep based on just age alone. Your sleep needs might differ from these recommendations since they are based on what the average person requires.

Note: Just because someone can get by with less sleep than this does not mean they should. Your sleep quality is not solely determined by how rested you feel or how well you can function—so keep that in mind as we proceed.

The Centers for Disease Control (CDC, 2002) recommends the following nightly hours of sleep per age group:

- children (aged 6–12): 8–12 hours
- teenagers (aged 13–18): 8–10 hours
- adults (aged 18–64): 7–9 hours
- seniors (aged 65 and older): 7–8 hours

Adults with less than seven hours of sleep per night are more vulnerable to health risks. On the other hand, there are no proven risks associated with sleeping more than nine hours on some occasions.

Again, these are only recommendations. Your personal conditions might require you to get more sleep than this. Sleep needs can be influenced by pregnancy, previous sleep deprivation, sleep quality, and how your sleep patterns change with age. For example, someone pregnant might be sleeping less than usual due to changes in hormones and physical discomfort. This means they might need more hours to make up for it.

To access your personal sleep needs, ask yourself these questions:

- Are you happy and productive with the rest you're currently getting?
- Do you have other health concerns that might influence your sleep needs?
- Are you expending much energy on an average day?
- How much alertness does your daily routine require? Do you feel sufficiently vigilant with how much sleep you're getting?
- Do you have a history of sleep disturbances?
- Do you rely on caffeine or energy drinks to keep you going?
- Do you sleep in if you are not bound to a specific schedule?

These questions won't give you an exact answer, but they will help you determine if your needs are being met. You can use these questions at any point to reassess how well you're sleeping.

Changing how long we rest is not the only way to improve our sleep. However, it is often the first step in developing better sleeping patterns.

THE SCIENCE OF SLEEP

For a long time, people believed—and often still do—that sleep is a period of inactivity and dormancy. Modern research has shown that this is not the case. In truth, sleep is a biological function that's essential to our survival, much like breathing or digestion. During it, our brains perform tasks to ensure we stay functional.

Sleep Cycles

Sleep can be broken up into a series of cycles. On average, people go through five or six of them each night. Each cycle consists of different stages, all with their own functions and processes. The duration of these cycles changes over the course of the night. Earlier on, cycles are shorter, averaging around 70–100 minutes each. Later in the night, though, cycles become longer, averaging about 90–120 minutes each.

Understanding the sleep cycle can help you optimize your behavior and habits. It can help you, as well, to figure out the best time to wake up or go to sleep and offer insight into where things go wrong.

The Stages of Sleep

The sleep cycle has four separate stages. These stages can be categorized as either rapid eye movement (REM) sleep or non-REM sleep.

Non-REM sleep stages make up most of the cycle. They are what progress us from wakefulness to rest and back. These phases are where most of the beneficial processes take place. During non-REM sleep, your body will:

- build muscle and bone
- repair and regenerate damaged tissue
- strengthen the immune system

REM sleep is characterized by increased brain activity and quick, darting eye movements. During this phase, your brain activity comes close to what it is while you're awake. For this reason, you can dream while in this stage of sleep. Dreams can also occur in other stages, but not as commonly or intensely as in REM sleep. It's believed that this phase influences cognitive abilities like memory, creativity, and learning.

Altogether, a single sleep cycle will look like this:

Stage 1.

During this phase, the body goes from being awake to being asleep. Your breathing becomes slower, and your muscles relax. You might dip in and out of consciousness during this time or experience the sensation of falling. It's common to feel your muscles jerk or to wake up very easily. Often, people who wake up here can recall images and sounds. If you wake frequently during this period, it might feel like you haven't slept at all.

Stage 2.

This is a stretch of light sleep. Here, your body relaxes even more, and the brain prepares for deep sleep. Now, breathing, heart rate, and body temperature will decrease even more, and all eye movements will stop. This stage is marked by slower brain activity with short spikes of heightened activity. These spikes are called sleep spindles, believed to be the brain storing memories or shutting down senses.

Stage 3.

This is known as deep sleep or slow-wave sleep. This is where most of our functional rest comes from. Biological processes like heart rate and breathing are at their slowest here. Brain waves slow down into delta waves. Delta waves are the slowest frequency brain waves and are often associated with healing and restoration. It's a lot harder to wake someone when they're in deep sleep. You'll likely feel groggy and disoriented if you do get awoken here. Interestingly, the duration of this stage changes with each cycle. It lasts longer earlier in the night and begins getting shorter as you get closer to the morning. This is also one of the stages that are most impacted by age. Older adults spend less time in stage 3 than their younger counterparts.

Stage 4.

This is REM sleep. During this stage, brain activity, heart rate, and blood pressure increase. At the same time, most of your muscles become paralyzed temporarily to limit physical reactions to brain activity. Like deep sleep, the duration of REM sleep changes. At the start of the night, REM sleep is relatively short (approximately 10 minutes). As the night progresses, REM sleep lasts longer.

Factors That Influence the Sleep Cycle

Sleep is a complex process, and it's managed by neurotransmitters (nervous system cells that transfer messages and signals between other cells). Anything that influences those neurotransmitters will also influence your sleep cycles. These influences include:

- **Alcohol:** A drink before bed can help someone fall asleep but reduces their time in deep sleep. While it might help you drift off, it ultimately leads to a lesser quality sleep that is more easily interrupted.
- **Caffeine:** This is a stimulant and makes it harder for your brain to relax when it comes time to go to sleep. It can also affect how well your brain responds to certain neurotransmitters. For example, it impedes the absorption of melatonin (the hormone responsible for making you feel sleepy). Both factors lead to worse quality sleep and difficulties falling and staying asleep.
- **Medications:** Certain medications contain chemical compounds that can lead to higher agitation and reduced sleep. Pseudoephedrine (a chemical found in certain decongestants), alpha-blockers, certain antidepressants (predominantly those that are listed as selective serotonin-reuptake inhibitors—SSRIs), corticosteroids, and pain medications that contain

caffeine are all examples. Do not stop taking prescribed medication without consulting a doctor. Some medications must be weaned off, while others might be prescribed for potentially life-altering conditions.

- **Smoking:** Those who smoke heavily have been found to wake up more frequently during the night and are known for having short periods of REM sleep. This can be a result of nicotine cravings.

- **Temperature:** The body always maintains a well-balanced temperature, even during sleep. While asleep, your body temperature is lowered. When you enter REM sleep, this regulation slackens somewhat, which can lead to interruptions in your sleep if you're in an environment that's too hot or too cold.

- **Age:** Our sleeping patterns change as we age. The most significant of these is the effect on REM sleep. Infants spend much longer in the REM stage and enter it sooner than adults. Older adults have shorter REM stages than younger adults. Similarly, children experience longer periods of deep sleep than adults. Sleepwalking is more common in children for this reason since it occurs during deep sleep stages.

- **Recent sleep patterns:** The quality of your current sleep patterns will influence your future sleep needs. It will also affect how the brain regulates sleep stages. Those who have recently experienced irregular sleep are more likely to experience irregular cycles the next time they go to bed.

- **Sleep disorders:** A history of sleep disorders will influence your sleep cycles. If you have conditions like sleep apnea or restless leg syndrome, you're more likely to wake up during the night.

INSOMNIA

What Is It?

The Sleep Foundation defines insomnia as "a sleep disorder characterized by difficulty with falling asleep, staying asleep, or both." (Suni, 2023b). Other definitions extend this to include consistently waking up earlier than you should and not being able to fall back asleep.

Put plainly; insomnia can present in different ways. Experts generally distinguish types of insomnia based on two key things: time and cause.

Time

On the one hand, there is acute or chronic insomnia. This differentiates types of insomnia based on how long it persists.

Acute means short-term and includes insomnia that lasts for a few days or weeks up to three months. If it lasts over three months, it becomes chronic insomnia (sometimes called insomnia disorder). Acute presentations tend to come from external influences like stress or changes in lifestyle and might not come with pronounced daytime side effects.

Chronic insomnia refers to sleep disruptions that last for an extended period. For insomnia to qualify as chronic, it must occur at least three days a week for more than three months.

Chronic insomnia is often linked to worsening symptoms. People with it often report feeling distressed by their symptoms and experience more pronounced daytime effects of the disorder.

Cause

Now, in this differentiation, different types of insomnia are caused by, well, different things.

Primary insomnia is understood as sleep disturbances that are unrelated to any other health condition. In this case, it is caused by external, dynamic influences like stress, life events, or personal experiences. It can also come from lifestyle influences like diet and exercise or habits like napping and using your phone before sleeping. This type of insomnia can persist long after that influence is gone.

On the other hand, secondary insomnia occurs because of another health condition or sleep disorder. For example, insomnia can be caused by sleep apnea, chronic pain, or as a side-effect of certain medications to treat other health issues. In these cases, sleep disturbances are a symptom or side-effect of the primary condition.

What Causes Insomnia?

A variety of influences can bring on insomnia. There is no one identifiable cause. These causes can also contribute to the severity of your symptoms. On that note, let's go over some common reasons.

- **Stress:** Worries regarding work, school, health, finances, and so on can make it challenging to get a decent night's rest. You can, quite literally, lose sleep over them. Stressful events like losing a loved one or traumatic experiences can further contribute to your overall stress and lead to insomnia. Stress influences how your brain responds to various stimuli. It often triggers your built-in stress response (fight-or-flight), prioritizing alertness over rest.

- **Schedules:** Your body runs on an internal clock called the circadian rhythm. This system uses an internal rhythm to regulate things like hunger and sleepiness. Disruptions to it can lead to all sorts of unpleasant issues like insomnia. Something that can disrupt this rhythm includes traveling to a different time zone, having odd hours for work shifts that make you work late or rise early, and having an irregular daily schedule. It can be further influenced by the quality of the light in your environment and how well you've slept recently.

- **Poor sleep habits and hygiene:** Our habits and regular routines influence how our bodies function. An irregular sleep schedule, diet, stimulation before bed, an uncomfortable sleep environment, or daytime naps can all affect how easily you fall asleep at night. On top of this, the light from computer screens, TVs, and cell phones can influence your internal clock, making it harder for your brain to tell when it's time to go to sleep.

- **Eating before bed:** Anything other than a light snack before sleep can contribute to your insomnia. Our metabolism is a primary biological function, and it involves a lot of complex processes. Eating before bed means these processes run while we try to shut down for the night. A full stomach can also cause discomfort while lying down, leading to symptoms like heartburn or acid reflux.

- **Mental health conditions:** Your mental health influences many things, including sleep quality. Disorders like anxiety, depression, or PTSD can make it difficult to fall asleep. They cause mental excitement, meaning your mind doesn't quiet down enough for you to doze off. Insomnia also worsens the mental health disorders that caused it in the first place, meaning it will likely lead to deteriorating mental health and, as a result, worsening insomnia.

- **Physical health conditions:** Several physical health issues have been identified as potential causes, including chronic pain, asthma, gastroesophageal reflux disease (GERD), thyroid dysfunctions, and diabetes. Anything that causes pain or discomfort will likely disrupt your sleep in some way or another. Physical health issues can also lead to specific needs that involve insufficient sleep. These can include, for example, needing to wake up for medicine at a particular time or having to go to the bathroom frequently.

- **Medications:** As mentioned previously, medications can contribute to sleep disruptions. This can be due to side effects. Many medications cause drowsiness and lethargy during the day, leading to decreased activity. Stopping certain medications can also lead to insomnia through withdrawal or changing how your body regulates hormones.

- **Other sleep disorders:** Insomnia is not the only sleep disorder by a long shot, even though it is the most common one. Other sleep disorders like sleep apnea, restless leg syndrome, sleep paralysis, and sleepwalking can all disrupt your sleep and affect the quality of it. In the long run, these disruptions can lead to insomnia.
- **Age:** Older people are more likely to have insomnia than younger people. Again, as we age, our sleep cycles change. The older you are, the less time you spend in deep sleep or REM sleep. This means it's easier to wake up. Older individuals are also more vulnerable to health concerns, making them more susceptible to sleep problems. At the same time, we tend to become less active with age. Decreased activity means more naps and less energy expenditure, which can influence how well—or poorly—we sleep.

Symptoms

Insomnia is a multifaceted condition. While disrupted sleep is its most prominent symptom, it's not the only one. Other symptoms are

- having trouble falling or staying asleep
- waking up earlier than planned or desired
- resistance against going to bed
- fatigue and lethargy during the day
- irritability, anxiety, and other mood changes

- gastrointestinal symptoms like nausea or stomachaches
- poor focus, memory, and concentration
- slower reflexes and reaction times
- worry or concern over going to sleep or not getting enough sleep
- relying on medications or substances to fall asleep
- headaches, particularly tension headaches
- malaise (feeling generally unwell)
- trouble with work, school, or socializing

Risk Factors for Developing Insomnia

Statistics have shown that certain groups of people are at a higher risk of experiencing insomnia symptoms. These risk factors are

- being assigned female at birth
- being older
- poor socioeconomic status
- chronic medical conditions that cause discomfort or pain
- other sleep disorders
- experiencing mental health issues
- being a light sleeper
- a history of substance abuse
- living in an unsafe environment or not feeling safe in your environment
- an irregular daily schedule
- experiencing stress

Please note that these risk factors do not mean you have insomnia. They mean you are statistically more likely to have insomnia than someone without these risk factors. Furthermore, they do not disqualify other sleep disorders or health issues. So, if you think you have insomnia based on your experiences and these risk factors, speak to a doctor to eliminate more serious problems.

INSOMNIA MYTHS

There are many untrue and misleading beliefs about insomnia out there. While they have been debunked, many of them are still circulating and thus affect the way people attempt to manage their insomnia. These beliefs might seem harmless but ultimately contribute to misinformation surrounding insomnia. Knowledge is power, and having the wrong information can make it incredibly hard to find the right way forward. Without further ado, let's go over some of these myths.

#1 There's Nothing You Can Do About It

This is just factually incorrect. There are multiple possible treatments and management strategies. They can range from formal medical treatment like medication and therapy to self-care techniques like sleep hygiene improvement.

#2 You Can Catch Up on Lost Sleep

There's a common misconception that you can recover lost sleep later when you have the time. This is primarily linked to not sleeping well during the week and making up for lost sleep over the weekend.

While it is true that sleep disruptions can change your sleep needs and will require you to sleep more, listen carefully: You cannot make up for lost sleep. Sleep is not a weekly quota to fill where you can add a few extra hours somewhere else to make up for what you missed. Instead, sleep turns into sleep debt, which needs to be paid back and recovered to reduce the burden of that debt.

At the same time, sleeping a little extra at odd times will only contribute to your insomnia in the long run. Sleeping longer on some days (or oversleeping) contributes to an irregular sleep schedule and disrupts your normal sleep-wake regulation. Catching up on missed sleep might make you feel better on that particular day, but ultimately adds to the problem.

#3 You Should Stay in Bed Until You Fall Asleep

A common belief is that you should stay in bed until you eventually drift off. This is not only ineffective in helping you fall asleep, but it's also actually counterproductive. The longer you lie there, the worse your anxiety will become and the harder it will be to fall asleep.

If this continues long enough, your brain will associate your bed with those unpleasant feelings. This means you remember those feelings every time you lie down, making it harder to relax the next time you want to try and sleep.

The golden rule for this is simple: If awake after 20 minutes, get up and do something relaxing. Once you feel tired again, lie down and try again.

#4 All Insomnia Medications Work the Same

Insomnia is a multifaceted condition that describes a variety of different experiences. Some people struggle with falling asleep, while others struggle to remain asleep. Some people experience both issues. As such, medications intended to counter them must be diverse and dynamic enough to address their various facets.

Something else to consider is that not everyone will react to medications in the same way. For example, if the goal of the medication is to help you fall asleep, it can do so by inducing sleep, mimicking hormones to make you feel drowsy, or acting as something to help you relax. For people who experience secondary insomnia, that medication can also include things that address the underlying sleep disturbances, like pain medication.

The point is that medication for insomnia can vary significantly in what it does, how it does it, and how it can apply to different cases.

#5 Good Sleep Is All About the Number of Hours

The amount of time you spend asleep is not the only indicator of its quality. How many hours you're getting is often easier to pinpoint and fix than some of the more complex things, so it's often one of the first things most people look at. You can get precisely the correct number of hours, and it won't matter if your sleep quality is still poor.

Ultimately, the important thing is the quality of sleep you're getting. The number of hours is only one aspect of that.

#6 Napping Helps Offset Insomnia

Daytime naps can help you recover energy or minimize the effects of sleep deprivation in a pinch, but it is only a temporary solution. Like sleeping in on weekends, napping is beneficial in the short term but potentially damaging in the long term. Inopportune naps affect your sleep-wake regulation and can make it harder to fall asleep at night since you might not feel drowsy.

Now, not all naps are bad. If you take naps, ensure they don't affect your regular sleep schedule and that you do not start relying on them to compensate for poor nighttime sleeping. They are not a replacement for proper sleep and cannot make up for not getting a good night's sleep. A good rule is to make sure you aren't sleeping past 3 p.m.

#7 Insomnia Is a Difficulty Falling Asleep

This myth comes from people's general understanding of what insomnia is. We know that difficulty falling asleep is one of insomnia's presentations, but it is not the only valid form of insomnia. The problem with this belief is that it ignores the other presentations. Someone who falls asleep quickly but frequently wakes up during the night is just as much an insom-niac as someone who lies in bed for an hour trying to nod off.

This myth is ultimately one of ignorance—but it can still be harmful. Many people think they do not have insomnia simply because they believe this myth and thus don't seek help for it.

#8 You'll Adjust to Getting Less Sleep

The idea here is that, after enough time, you can get used to not sleeping the recommended seven to nine hours and eventually adapt to getting less sleep. While this is true in that you'll "get used to it," it is not true that your body will adapt to it. Your sleep needs don't adjust to your schedule. You might get used to functioning in those conditions, but that need will remain unfulfilled. Like any unfulfilled need, this can have nasty conse-quences.

SLEEPING PILLS

Sleeping pills are medications a person can take to help them fall and stay asleep. These medications are known as sedative-hypnotics, a class of medications that lower the activity in a person's central nervous system. They can induce drowsiness, lessen anxiety, or even sedate the user.

Not all sleeping pills work the same. Some are used to manage thoughts and emotions that obstruct sleep. They help suppress some of the things that might be causing your insomnia or contributing to it. These pills often have drowsiness as a common side effect, making them useful as a sleeping aid.

Others bind to specific receptors in your brain to induce sleepiness. In short, they are often used to help a person fall asleep more easily. A third group mimics specific hormones to stimulate the body's natural sleep processes.

When sleep difficulties arise, our minds often go first to sleeping pills. They are convenient, as far as treatments go, and require minimal effort to use. All you need to do is take one before bed and wait for it to do its job.

On the surface, this is perfectly fine. However, sleeping pills should only be used as a temporary measure to fix your sleep schedule. It is not recommended for a person to take them regularly for a period longer than four weeks. They are a bridge you can use until your natural processes take over again. As such, they are there to help you overcome disruptions—not to be relied on forever.

Like all medications, sleeping pills come with risks and side effects. Most people tolerate them well enough when used correctly, but long-term or incorrect use can make them somewhat problematic.

The specific side effects of sleeping medications will vary depending on the brand and contents of the pill itself. Some common side effects include

- changes in appetite
- gastrointestinal symptoms like nausea, gas, stomach aches, constipation, and diarrhea
- dizziness and impaired balance
- dry mouth, eyes, and throat

- drowsiness throughout the day
- headaches
- trembling or shaking
- impaired mental function the next day, including brain fog, difficulty staying focused, and memory problems
- unusual, vivid dreams while asleep
- burning or tingling in the extremities

Long-Term Complications of Using Sleeping Pills

On top of the abovementioned side effects, sleeping pills also come with a list of long-term risks. Here are a few of those risks and how they might affect your life:

- **You can build up a tolerance to the medication.** The longer you use it, the more your body adapts to it. Soon, you'll need a higher dose to get the same effect. Higher doses often lead to more potent side effects, and you will eventually reach the upper limit of what is a safe dosage.
- **Daytime drowsiness.** Research suggests that the chemicals in certain medications can stay in your system for much longer than you might think. This can lead to impaired daily functioning, which can, in turn, have disastrous consequences when you consider actions like driving or childcare.
- **Erratic nighttime behavior or parasomnias.** Some sleeping pills can alter your behavioral patterns while asleep. This can result in odd behaviors, such as having entire conversations with people while still asleep. It

can also result in parasomnias (abnormal behavior while asleep) like sleep paralysis, nightmares, and sleepwalking. These are actions you have no control over. It can even make you forget what you did the previous night when you wake up the following day. In best-case scenarios, this can mean having a funny conversation with a loved one. In others, it can mean driving while asleep or using the stove to make food.

- **Increased risk of injury.** If you've ever taken a sleeping pill, you know they make you feel a little unsteady. If you leave the bed and walk while on them, you risk falling and getting hurt. One study found that hospital patients who took sleeping pills were up to four times more likely to fall than those who didn't. This can be a big issue if you are elderly or physically vulnerable.

- **Cancer and death.** Yes, you read that correctly. A pharmacological research study examined the long-term consequences of various sleeping pills in more than 10,000 cases (Kripke et al., 2012). This study concluded that patients who were using sleeping medications were three to five times more likely to die. The study also found an increased likelihood of cancer developing. Now, it's unclear exactly why these medications are linked to cancer. The increased mortality rate is easier to explain since most medications (sleeping pills or not) come with risks, but researchers don't know what to make of the potential cancer risks just yet.

- **You may become dependent on them.** Many sleeping pills are habit-forming, and many find they cannot simply stop taking them. When they do, they experience rebound insomnia. The best solution is to gradually wean the person off the medication until they can safely stop.

How to Wean Off Sleeping Pills

If you are taking sleeping pills and want to stop or have passed that recommended four-week time frame, I will offer you some tips for weaning off them.

First, it's recommended not to stop taking them cold turkey since this can result in rebound insomnia. This happens when a person experiences a reoccurrence of their insomnia symptoms after stopping a medication. Your body has learned to rely on the pills to signal when it should go to sleep; once you take that away, your body might not automatically restart its natural processes to replace those artificial signals, and as such, you might be stuck back at square one. Many cases of rebound insomnia can be worse than the original symptoms.

Furthermore, especially if you've been taking them for some time, you may experience physical withdrawal symptoms. Many of these medications are habit-forming or addictive and stopping them means your brain is no longer getting a supply of something it's come to depend on. Some common sleeping med withdrawal symptoms include anxiety, depression, restlessness, irritability, trembling, sweating, and confusion. In extreme cases, there might even be more severe effects like seizures and hallucinations.

To avoid this, taper off your sleeping medication. There are two ways to do this. One way is by gradually decreasing your dosage. For example, only take half a sleeping pill for a while. Alternatively, begin skipping certain nights of the medication. Start by only taking the medication six nights a week, then five, and so on, until you've stopped. Before doing any of this, however, consult a doctor or speak to a pharmacist, especially if you are taking prescription meds.

Secondly, begin changing your sleeping habits to replace the effect of the medication. If you've been on sleeping pills for a while, part of your sleeping routine will be to take a pill that will give your brain the necessary signals to sleep. To effectively stop them, you need to boost your brain's natural ability to do that independently. It's like breaking your arm and wearing a cast for several weeks; you need to rebuild the muscle and strength you lost while it was immobilized. You can almost consider these habits as rehab exercises for your sleeping centers.

Some things you can do to manage this are foregoing caffeine after a certain point in the day, not eating or drinking much in the hours before going to bed, exercising earlier in the day rather than later, avoiding television, computer, and cell phone screens before bed, and creating a sleep schedule (i.e., going to bed at the same time every night and waking up at the same time every morning). We'll discuss these habits in more detail later in Chapter 4. For now, know that you can transition from relying on sleeping pills to sleeping without them solely by optimizing your habits.

SLEEP SELF-ASSESSMENT

Online self-assessment tests will not be able to give you a diagnosis. However, they can help give you an idea of whether or not to see your doctor. Why? Because they offer an objective way of considering your experiences.

That said, do not make drastic changes to your lifestyle based on a self-assessment test, and certainly do not ignore concerning symptoms. If you are concerned enough to take a test online, it's probably worth seeing a doctor regardless, particularly if your symptoms persist.

There are several different tests you can do. Some measure your symptoms to gauge how likely you are to have insomnia. Others might measure your symptoms to determine how severe your insomnia is (or isn't). Look up "sleep self-assessment" on any search engine to find a few. I will also provide one below that you can do.

For each of the following questions, select one of the options that best represents your experiences over the past month. Keep track of your answers since they will be added together to create a score. The points for each option are as follows: a = 4, b = 3, c = 2, d = 1, and e = 0.

1. How long does it take you to fall asleep?

    a. 0–15 min
    b. 16–30 min
    c. 31–45 min
    d. 45–60 min
    e. More than 60 min

2. How long (in total) did you spend awake after waking up during the night?

    a. 0–15 min
    b. 16–30 min
    c. 31–45 min
    d. 45–60 min
    e. More than 60 min

3. How many nights a week do you experience insomnia symptoms?

    a. 0–1
    b. 2
    c. 3
    d. 4
    e. 5–7

4. How good is your quality of sleep?

    a. Very good
    b. Good
    c. Average
    d. Poor
    e. Very Poor

5. Has your sleep affected your relationships, mood, and energy?

    a. Not at all
    b. A little
    c. Moderately
    d. A good deal
    e. A lot

6. Has your sleep affected your focus and productivity?

    a. Not at all
    b. Very little
    c. Moderately
    d. A good deal
    e. A lot

7. How much trouble has your sleep caused you?

    a. None
    b. Very little
    c. A moderate amount
    d. A good amount
    e. A lot

8. How long have you been experiencing these issues?

    a. Less than one month
    b. 1–2 months
    c. 3–6 months
    d. 7–12 months
    e. More than one year

Add your points together. A score of less than 16 means you may have insomnia. The lower your score, the more symptoms of insomnia you have. The higher your score, the better your sleep is. That is not to say a score of 16 or higher means you don't have insomnia; it only means you have fewer expected symptoms and experiences.

Doctors often perform a similar screening when diagnosing insomnia. On top of this, they might also do a mental health check-up, conduct a sleep study, or ask you to keep a sleep journal to investigate possible causes or contributing factors.

2

IT STARTS WITH YOUR MINDSET

 Mind is a flexible mirror; adjust it to see a better world.

— AMIT RAY

WHAT IS MINDSET AND HOW DOES IT AFFECT YOUR SLEEP?

Mindset refers to how you approach life. It influences how you interact with yourself and the world around you, what you think and feel, and how you behave.

You might wonder why this is important or what mindset even has to do with sleep. Your mindset influences your behaviors and habits, which, in turn, impacts your sleep. Mindset also has a great deal of influence on mental health, which most certainly affects your sleep. In many ways, mindset can be the primary catalyst for our troubles, including those we have with rest.

A great deal of our experiences come down to mental toughness. Mental toughness refers to how well you can adapt to what life throws at you. It determines how you respond to anxiety, negative thoughts and feelings, and stress. Mental toughness is not about remaining untouched by these things but about maintaining the ability to persevere despite them. It is not about toughing out demanding situations and remaining aloof in the face of difficulty. It is about facing those difficulties and coming out on top. In other words, mental toughness is about your mindset and how you face life.

The right mindset will help you address and balance the issues contributing to your insomnia. It can help you manage anxiety, develop and maintain a good sleeping schedule, and give you the wherewithal to grow healthier habits.

FIXED VERSUS GROWTH MINDSET

When it comes to mindset, there are two main ones to discuss. The first is a fixed mindset. People with this mindset believe that their intelligence, creativity, and talents have been predetermined and are static. The second is a growth mindset. People with this mindset believe that intelligence and talent are skills that can be developed. In this case, they are not static but dynamic.

In other words, with a fixed mindset, you are limited to your natural abilities, but with a growth mindset, those abilities can be improved upon. With a fixed mindset, it's all about what you have, whereas with a growth mindset, it's about what you have the potential to be.

The main difference between the two for our purposes lies in how you handle situations. With a fixed mindset, people think of setbacks as failures and things to be avoided. On the other hand, someone with a growth mindset considers a setback as a challenge to overcome. Challenges may be tough for people with a fixed mindset because they might think they cannot overcome them. On the other hand, someone with a growth mindset will consider the problem and develop the abilities they need.

There is no quick fix for insomnia. Managing it will require time and dedication; even then, it takes trial and error to balance habits and routines. That's hard to do with a fixed mindset. When something doesn't work immediately, or a new thing you tried fails, you'll need that growth mindset to keep going. It's really all about changing the fixed "I can't sleep properly" into "I struggle to sleep, but there are things I can try, and I can ask for help." It's a slight difference but a meaningful one.

HOW MINDSET SHAPES YOUR LIFE

Our lives shape our mindset, which continues to shape our lives. It influences how we act, think, and react. It impacts a large portion of who we are. This is true for life in general, and it's also true for how we deal with insomnia. Let's now look at how a fixed and growth mindset might shape some essential aspects of your life:

With a fixed mindset, a person

- is resistant to change and skeptical of challenges
- values talent and ability over effort and persistence
- seeks approval
- views setbacks as failures
- lacks the motivation to make changes due to a belief that it won't contribute anything

With a growth mindset, a person

- embraces challenges and change
- values persistence and hard work over born ability
- seeks information and development
- views setbacks as temporary and learns from them
- is willing to try new things and explore new options

Our mindset can even contribute to our insomnia. Having a fixed mindset might make it easier to feel overwhelmed when faced with challenges. You might be more anxious or worried that you aren't up to scratch with a fixed mindset than with a growth mindset.

This, combined with your mindset making it challenging to adapt to new treatment strategies, can make insomnia ten times harder to manage. A big part of conquering it involves changing your habits and routines. This may require changing your way of thinking. These are things people with a fixed mindset find difficult. In many ways, a fixed mindset can sabotage your efforts before they have a chance.

Someone with a fixed mindset might see insomnia as something they were bound to end up with and something they can't do anything about. They might have a more challenging time learning how to manage it due to their resistance to change. In some cases, they might not consider themselves capable of learning new skills or being able to adjust to a new routine. Many view insomnia as a personal failure and, as such, feel reluctant to talk about it with others. Someone with a fixed mindset might think: "I'm high-strung and just don't sleep well. It's always been like that. It is what it is."

On the other hand, a growth mindset might put you on the right track. With it, you are more resilient when it comes to setbacks. When you believe you can grow and develop, you open yourself up to changing your habits for better outcomes. You might be more open to learning or trying new things. Indeed, with a growth mindset, you can change your lifestyle, learn new skills, and bounce back from relapses and failures. Someone with this mindset sees insomnia as an obstacle to overcome and not something they're doomed to endure for life. They would not consider changing their sleep to be an impossible task. Someone with a growth mindset might think: "I have trouble sleeping right now, but if I put in the work, I can learn to manage it and improve my sleep quality."

CHANGING YOUR MINDSET—PUTTING IT IN PRACTICE

If you want to explore shifting your mindset, I encourage you to do more in-depth research. There are beneficial exercises online that can help you make the necessary changes. To give you some tips here and now, though, try out the following:

- Incorporate "yet" into your thoughts and beliefs. For example, "I can't do this yet."
- Find value in the journey. Instead of focusing solely on the problem and solutions, consider your journey. Insomnia is difficult, but it's also a process of learning healthier habits and changing things that aren't working.
- Replace negative, pessimistic thoughts with more positive and realistic ones. For example, turn "This is impossible" into "I can overcome this with some effort."
- Embrace the challenges that come with the journey. It isn't always easy; instead of avoiding difficulties, face them head-on and learn from them. Setbacks aren't something to avoid. They are, in fact, an inevitability, and accepting this truth makes it easier to cope when we experience setbacks.

Here are some sleep-specific changes to your mindset that you can put into practice:

- Anxiety about losing sleep is a significant contributor to insomnia. We worry about why we can't sleep, what will happen tomorrow, and if we're losing control, and as a result, we agonize over the sleep we aren't getting. Instead, experts recommend accepting that some nights will be worse than others and letting go of the anxieties surrounding those bad nights. Instead of putting your energy into worrying over your lost sleep, put it into something that might help you fall asleep, like doing some breathing exercises to relax or getting up and doing something else until you're ready to try again.

- See each night as a new, separate night. As humans, we recognize patterns and then base our behavior on them. In the case of insomnia, we often take the fact that we haven't slept well the past few nights as an indicator that we won't sleep well tonight. Doing this creates an expectation that we won't sleep, influencing how we behave when we go to bed. We close ourselves off from the possibility of sleep by accepting that tonight will be just as bad as last night. In a way, we create a sort of self-fulfilling prophecy. Seeing each night as a new night reduces our anxiety about sleep, which makes it easier to fall asleep. If you fall into this trap, though it might sound simple or silly, try thinking, "It might be bad—but it might also not be." At the same time, don't let the previous night influence your routine and sleeping schedule. Also, don't try to go to bed early.

Going to bed before you're tired will make it harder to sleep.

- Put your worries about tomorrow aside. In the modern age, it's tough to disconnect. Our phones and internet access keep us connected to the world. We keep them close in case someone needs us; we check our emails before bed and scroll through social media because it's always right there at our fingertips. This makes it incredibly hard to shut down for sleep. But the truth is, nothing needs your attention right now, and everything will be there when you wake up. Try turning your phone and computer off after a specific time of the evening. You can even leave them in another room. This also applies to other work-related things, school projects, or anything else interfering with your rest, like TV.

- Prioritize your health. Many believe "One all-nighter won't hurt," or "I'm good on six hours of sleep." You are not. Prioritize your health and well-being by taking clear measures, like getting enough sleep.

- Change your attitude toward sleep. It is a good use of your time. Too often, I encounter people who consider sleeping something that takes up hours they could use to do something else, and that's an incredibly damaging mindset. Sleep is important. It heals you, recovers energy, and sets you up for productivity. Ignoring it will inevitably lead to having fewer hours to do those seemingly important things. If you think like this, remind yourself that sleep is not a waste of time but something that improves your health and well-being.

- Manage your thoughts. We already know that thoughts and feelings contribute to both insomnia and our mindset. So, instead of letting them drag you under, try something new by applying some mindfulness to your thinking. Learn to recognize the thoughts that influence your sleeping issues. Label them by reframing them into "I notice I have the thought that..." This creates some distance between you and that thought, so it won't affect you as much. Once you've done this, treat that thought with compassion. Try to understand why you have it and reassure yourself that it's okay to have that thought before ultimately letting it go.

- Let go of expectations. Many times, we try too hard to fall asleep. Stick with me here for a second. We get so desperate to sleep that we start trying everything. When those things don't work, we get desperate and try harder. This is simply counterproductive. The more pressure we put on ourselves to fall asleep, the more unlikely it will become. Instead, try to depressurize the process. Let go of some of the expectations. If you don't sleep, you don't. Stop trying and just let it happen. Practice some relaxation exercises like deep breathing to let go of the expectations you might have.

LETTING GO OF NEGATIVE THOUGHTS

You know that negative thoughts at bedtime affect your sleep, but did you know that your daytime thoughts have the same effect? One study found a correlation between daytime thoughts and sleep outcomes (Galbiati et al., 2018). It suggests a difference between the type of negative thoughts we may have, mainly distinguishing them into either rumination or worry. Worry relates to concerns about the future, while rumination relates to repetitive thoughts about negative thoughts and experiences. The study found that worry led to waking up more frequently during the night, less total sleep time, less REM sleep, and overall decreased sleep quality. Meanwhile, rumination affects sleep quality and sleep latency (how quickly someone falls asleep).

Worry and rumination are not inherently bad; it's how we manage them that matters. Worrying can even be healthy. It lets us identify potential problems and come up with solutions in advance. Furthermore, it helps us plan and prepare. In contrast, it becomes unhealthy when it leads to uncontrollable spirals that make the issue worse than it was. For example, a healthy worry might be, "Am I unhealthy? I should try to be healthier," while an unhealthy worry is, "Am I unhealthy? What if I get so sick that I can't work anymore? What will I do then—will I be able to take care of myself?"

How to Quiet Negative Thoughts

Often, our first reaction to negative thoughts is to engage them or suppress them. Engaging with them leads to spiraling and suppressing them makes them worse. We cannot think ourselves out of negative thoughts, especially when trying to fall asleep.

A healthy way to deal with them is to learn how to identify them, find out where they come from or what caused them, question whether they're accurate, and then reframe them into something more helpful. This is a cognitive restructuring process used in many kinds of therapies to deal with negative thoughts. When doing this, you guide your mind through disconnecting from unrealistic negative thought patterns that aren't healthy. When you do this, you learn how to reduce the impact of thoughts on the rest of your life.

So, if you're faced with negative thoughts that are keeping you awake, try some of these methods:

- **Distract yourself with something trivial or meaningless.** Try to recount meaningless lists or run through trivial mental exercises. Aim for something of no real importance that will not engage your mind to the point of excitement. Your mind can latch onto this so it doesn't start spiraling into negativity. For example, list all the things you would add onto a private jet or think up dishes you would include in a celebratory banquet if you were ever given a Nobel prize. Alternatively, try mental puzzles like counting backward by seven (i.e., 1000, 993, 986, etcetera).
- **Keep a journal of the thoughts that are keeping you awake.** Objectivity is incredible and hard to maintain. The more time you spend with thoughts, the less perspective you have. Seeing words on paper forces some distance and often shifts your point of view. Having everything written down can help you achieve some objectivity. It's also therapeutic to get everything out instead of letting it swirl inside you. If you cannot

fall asleep, get up and empty your head onto a piece of paper before trying again.

- **Do some deep breathing.** Deep breathing triggers our natural relaxation responses and reduces stress levels. It's a great way to force some relaxation into your body. Counting your breaths also gives your mind something to focus on. Try four counts in and six counts out. Alternatively, try the 4-7-8 method, inhaling for four counts, holding for seven, and then exhaling for eight counts.
- **Create a routine where you perform the same few actions in the same order before lying down to sleep.** Keep these actions consistent and make sure they are relaxing. Eventually, your brain will learn to associate them with going to sleep; just performing them will help you enter the right state of being.

Everyone is different and finding things that work for you might take some time. Don't be afraid to try things out or have some of them not work as well as expected. Experiment with different exercises or tactics and change how you do something if it doesn't work. You can also look up other strategies if none are right for you.

TOO IMPERFECT TO FALL ASLEEP

Do you consider yourself a perfectionist? If so, this section is for you. Perfectionism can be described as a drive to ensure that everything is perfect or flawless, including yourself and how others perceive you. It drives you to fulfill impossible standards. It is characterized by a fear of failure, procrastination, goal-focused thinking, overly critical, and unrealistic expectations. In some cases, it leads to a person only participating in things guaranteed to be successful.

Research suggests that there is a link between perfectionism and sleep disturbances. Many people who identify as perfectionists develop untrue beliefs and thought patterns surrounding sleep. This can be due to the anxiety that keeps them from sleep or because they sacrifice sleep in the pursuit of perfection. To cope with that, they develop unhealthy sleeping habits, like working late into the night, discounting the value of sleep, taking naps to circumvent sleep deprivation symptoms, or harboring sleep-related anxiety.

Perfectionists try to control their lives to achieve the best results. If something doesn't work, they'll double their efforts to make it work. As we know, the more you try to fall asleep, the harder it will be. This frustrates the perfectionist. For them, the outcome of not being able to sleep, no matter how hard they try, is a failure on their part. Since they are already predisposed toward a fear of failure or performance anxiety regarding outcomes, this makes insomnia harder for them to manage.

While setbacks are hard for the average person, a perfectionist takes it extra hard. To them, there is no temporary setback. They tend to have an all-or-nothing approach. Something is right or wrong, good or bad, successful or not. This mindset adds to the stress they feel in their everyday lives and extends to their sleep.

So, what can you do about this? The first step is to embrace your imperfections. You are human, and that comes with having flaws. As frustrating as it might be, you must learn to embrace these things about yourself. You do not have to be perfect or flawless to be worth it. To do that, try the following things:

- **Find positives in your flaws.** As cliché as it sounds, find a silver lining. Learn to stop viewing yourself through that all-or-nothing lens. What you perceive as a flaw is more complex and can even be beautiful, depending on how you look at it. Try seeing each flaw in a new light. Find the gray areas. Then, let those facts form your opinion.

- **Be inspired by art.** If ever there is something that immortalizes imperfection, it is art. You'll find flaws if you truly look at art (whether it's paintings, tapestries, sculptures, or any other form of creative expression). Some even have them deliberately included. The concept of perfect imperfection has been propagated in art for centuries, yet we still celebrate its beauty. If we can accept the imperfections in art, we can accept the imperfections in ourselves.

- **Recognize that your imperfections are normal and that they are what makes you human.** You are not a robot. People are flawed; it's what makes us the complex, capable creatures we are. If this is difficult for you, remember that seemingly flawless people are also flawed. Stop trying to hide your quirks and irregularities. Learn to accept them as part of who you are. Note, however, that this is not a carte blanche permission to disregard valid criticisms and ignore the need to work on toxic traits. Self-improvement is not a bad thing.

- **Surround yourself with positives.** What we surround ourselves with influences our entire mindset. If you immerse yourself in negatives, you'll become more negative. Likewise, if you surround yourself with overly critical people, you will become that. On the other hand, if you surround yourself with positivity and support, you'll feel freer.
- **Embrace a flow state rather than perfection.** We tend to perceive perfection as a requirement for meeting a goal and build our processes around that. Instead, treat perfection as a goal so that it becomes a motivator and something to work toward rather than an impediment to the process.
- **Use your imperfections to serve you and others.** Accepting your imperfections is difficult, but you can use that experience to help others do the same. At the same time, many of our perceived imperfections aren't all that bad. We learn to view them as imperfect because of how we believe perfection to be. But our imperfections can be useful once we remove them from that context. Find ways to play to your strengths, even if that includes applying your so-called imperfections.
- **Talk to others.** Knowing you're not the only one struggling with this can help a lot. You can also ask other people's opinions to broaden your perspective. It can help you learn how to see things differently.

You might wonder why it's necessary to do any of this. Learning to love your imperfections means you won't feel as much pressure to change them. It lets you be at peace with who you are and removes some of the expectations you might struggle with. That kind of self-security will help you let go of the tensions that might keep you awake at night.

3

STRESS LESS, SLEEP BETTER

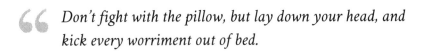 *Don't fight with the pillow, but lay down your head, and kick every worriment out of bed.*

— ELIE WIESEL

WHAT IS STRESS?

Verywell Mind defines stress as "any type of change that causes physical, emotional, or psychological strain" (Scott, 2022). It can also be defined as the body's natural response to a perceived threat, pressuring situations, or notable events. In short, it is our natural response to things that require immediate attention.

We use the term stress to describe the feeling we get when our body triggers its natural stress response (also known as fight-or-flight). This response is, in part, a survival mechanic. When activated, it changes the body and brain to assist you in a dangerous situation. This response prepares you to either run away or fight. It does this by increasing your heart rate, blood pressure, and blood oxygenation. It also makes you more alert. In short, it redirects natural resources to those systems that will help you survive.

Stress is a natural process. It isn't necessarily bad for you, but it becomes that when you are exposed to it continuously without time to rest and recuperate. Stress is meant to be temporary. Once the threat has passed, the body is meant to relax and return to normal, but that doesn't happen when we are constantly exposed to the things that cause us stress in the first place.

What Causes It?

Everyone experiences stress differently, and its causes can vary drastically from person to person. The things that stress one person might not affect someone else. To determine the causes of your stress, you'll need to take the time to evaluate your life. Try to pinpoint when you feel stressed and then use those moments to identify the stressors that triggered or contributed to it.

Some common stressors include

- experiencing a natural disaster
- living with a chronic health condition
- having your life or safety threatened by an accident or illness

- familial troubles like divorce, conflict, or abuse
- seeing loved ones suffer
- finances
- relationships
- having a high-risk career
- an unhealthy work-life balance
- being faced with discrimination or harassment
- exposure to something you fear, like heights or spiders
- mental health difficulties

Anything that triggers a reaction from you can qualify as a stressor.

Types of Stress

There are three types of stress.

The first is **acute stress**. The word acute is used to refer to short-term experiences. Acute stress is a temporary stress reaction to an immediate stimulus. It's what you experience during or after an accident (or near-accident) or a roller coaster ride. In cases like the latter, it can even be thrilling or exciting.

This kind of stress is common, and it's the one we experience the most. It usually has a short onset and passes relatively quickly. Now, this kind of stress is not necessarily unhealthy. It can be beneficial since it provides your body with a way to develop responses to stressful events. Note, however, that severe acute stress is an entirely different matter. If acute stress comes from a disturbing event (something life-threatening) or the stress response is especially strong, it could lead to PTSD and phobias.

The second is **episodic acute stress**. This is when you have frequent episodes of acute stress. Each episode is an acute stress experience, i.e., a short-term stress response in reaction to certain situations. This is common in people with jobs with high-stress moments like law enforcement or emergency situations. It is also common in people with anxiety.

In the case of extreme stress, episodic stress can have serious mental health consequences.

The third type is **chronic stress**. This comes from experiencing higher levels of stress for extended periods. This is not the same as episodic stress, where a person frequently experiences stress responses. In this case, the person is exposed to constant, inescapable stress, or stress that never ends. This can happen in cases where people are constantly exposed to a stressor, for example, a bad marriage or high-stress career.

Chronic stress often leads to health complications since the body never entirely switches off the stress response or engages the relaxation response. It can lead to anxiety, heart problems, high blood pressure, and sleep disturbances.

All three can contribute to insomnia in different ways. Recognizing which one you're dealing with can help you identify management strategies.

Signs and Symptoms

Stress can affect different parts of your being. As such, I've organized the common symptoms of stress into three categories: physical, mental, and behavioral.

Common physical symptoms of stress include

- headaches
- muscle tension and pain
- chest pain
- fatigue or undue tiredness
- changes in libido
- gastrointestinal issues like nausea, upset stomach, stomach pain, and acid reflux
- heartburn
- changes in appetite
- sweaty palms
- more frequent infections and illness
- trembling or shaking
- heart palpitations or racing heart

Common mental symptoms of stress include

- anxiety
- restlessness
- lack of motivation and interest
- feeling overwhelmed
- irritability
- irrational or unprovoked anger

- depression

Common behavioral symptoms of stress include

- eating more or less than normal
- lashing out at the slightest inconvenience
- substance abuse, particularly increased smoking or drinking
- social withdrawal and self-isolation
- exercising less or being less active
- difficulty sleeping

If you do not experience any of these symptoms, that doesn't mean you aren't stressed. Stress presents differently in different people. These are only some of the most reported symptoms.

How Stress Affects Your Health

Stress isn't necessarily bad. It is our body's way of reacting to certain situations. It exists to keep us safe and protect us from bodily harm. It's how we manage it and how frequently we are exposed to it that makes it bad.

Think about it this way: Stress isn't just a casual reaction to stimulus. It's a complex biological process. It's accompanied by changes in our hormones and biological functions, which is why stress is so damaging in the long run; it changes our normal functioning. These changes aren't meant to be permanent. They're meant to be something temporary, something reversible.

When fight-or-flight is triggered, it releases stress hormones. These hormones deliver signals to other parts of the body to increase oxygenation, redirect blood flow, and increase alertness. This allows us to be more aware of our surroundings and increase our odds of survival by making us better runners and fighters. To do this, however, those resources are pulled from other systems. While the stress response is active, it shuts down the processes that manage reproductive and growth hormones, the immune system, and digestion. This doesn't have significant consequences in the short term, but I'm sure you can see why this might be bad in the long run. We need that stress response to calm down so resources can be returned to those systems.

At the same time, the stress response places strain on the heart, lungs, and musculoskeletal structure. For one, your muscles tense up. This happens because your body prepares for action and to defend against injuries. With acute stress, this can happen suddenly, without warning, and then be rereleased relatively quickly. These quick changes can be incredibly uncomfortable. In the case of chronic stress, this tension is maintained for extended periods, leading to muscle aches, tension headaches, jaw pain, and back pain.

Secondly, our breathing patterns change when we're stressed. Indeed, our breathing becomes faster and shallower, and this is due to the body's need for higher levels of oxygen. The body usually maintains a strict balance of oxygen and carbon dioxide in the blood. When breathing changes during periods of stress, that balance is thrown off. You may feel short of breath or experience chest tightness. This might not be much of an issue for most people and can easily be remedied with some slow, deep breaths. However, if you have an unrelated breathing issue (like asthma), this can cause other breathing problems.

Finally, the heart. The cardiovascular system consists of two main elements: the heart and the blood vessels. They work together, moving blood throughout the body to transport oxygen to the areas that need it. Both parts experience significant changes under the stress response. The heart starts pumping faster and harder while the blood vessels dilate. This means higher blood pressure and more strain experienced by the cardiovascular system than normal. Chronic stress means this system is experiencing higher strain for extended periods of time and can lead to higher blood pressure and an increased risk of suffering a heart attack or stroke.

If that isn't enough, other long-term effects of stress include

- reproductive health issues (like erectile dysfunction, irregular menstruation, fertility issues, low libido, etc.)
- gastrointestinal symptoms
- hormonal imbalances
- nervous system regulation dysfunction
- declining mental health

Stress is so commonplace that we forget how harmful it can be, and that's not even mentioning how it affects sleep.

THE LINK BETWEEN STRESS AND INSOMNIA

Stress and sleep are considered reciprocal systems, which means they influence each other. High stress levels can lead to sleep disturbances, while lack of sleep worsens stress.

There are many reasons why this happens. For starters, stress keeps our minds running. It sharpens our awareness and encourages physical changes which are incompatible with sleep. For example, during sleep, the heart rate slows and blood pressure decreases, while the opposite happens when you're stressed.

Another significant contributor to this cycle is the hormonal changes that come with stress. Stress hormones are released when fight-or-flight is activated. One of these hormones is cortisol, which increases your alertness. This same hormone is also used in the sleep-wake cycle. It's highest in the mornings to shake off sleep and encourage wakefulness but decreases significantly at night to prepare for sleep. If these levels rise with stress, it messes with the natural regulation of the sleep-wake cycle.

Research has shown that people with insomnia have higher levels of cortisol in the evenings. Whether this is the cause of insomnia or a side-effect is still unclear.

At the same time, your sleep quality affects your stress levels. Sleep itself affects your mood and emotional regulation, after all. Poor sleep can lead to more negative emotions and higher reactivity to those emotions. This often leads to stressful situations and, thus, increased stress overall. Poor sleep also has physical effects that contribute to our stress sensitivity, like higher cortisol levels, inflammation, and decreased neurological regulation.

All the details aside, stress leads to poor sleep, which leads to more stress and even poorer sleep. This is known as the stress-sleep cycle, and the good news is that you can break free from it —seriously.

HOW TO BREAK THE STRESS-SLEEP CYCLE

One way to break the cycle is to address either one of its components. You can focus entirely on managing stress or on improving your sleep. However, the best way is to do both. By targeting both, you won't have to compensate for the other. That said, stress is the easier of the two to take in hand, so most of the techniques I discuss will focus on that. Once your stress levels even out, you'll feel that sleep improves naturally. Many of these methods are also known to improve sleep simultaneously.

Anything that helps you destress and relax will help here. It's nearly impossible to remove stress from your life entirely—certainly not in today's world—but you can control how you manage it. Part of that means limiting your exposure to stressors where possible. If you know something causes stress, ask yourself if you can avoid it. This isn't always possible; we can't quit our jobs just because they stress us out. However, if you can limit your exposure to specific stressors, do that. If you can't, the next best approach is to learn how to minimize the effects of their influence on your life.

Here are a few ways to do that:

- **Say no to late nights.** Don't put yourself in situations where you'll be out or up doing something late into the night. An easy way to do this is to pick a bedtime (e.g., 11 p.m.) and then shift your schedule to ensure you are in bed by that time. This might mean making changes to ensure you are home well before then, so you'll have time to get ready to wind down and sleep.
- **Destress during the day.** If you've identified the stressors in your life, you can start working toward managing them. Add time into your schedule to destress. This can mean taking a walk after work, reading, pursuing a hobby, or meditating during the day. It can also mean taking five minutes to breathe and depressurize after a stressful event.
- **Manage your sleep.** Become the manager of your sleep routine. Make it a procedure and a habit. An hour before your chosen bedtime, begin quieting down and getting ready to sleep. Set a simple routine to help you slip into the right headspace. Fill this time with relaxing activities like gentle stretching, drinking a cup of tea, or reading a calming book.
- **Put away the technology and devices.** Switch off your phone, shut the laptop, and turn off the TV. There are better times to answer messages, scroll through social media, or check your emails. The light given off by your devices influences your sleep-wake cycle. Furthermore, they provide access to stimulating information. It's hard to shut down when the whole world is at our fingertips.

If you're concerned about being unreachable, ask yourself if you are needed or if the things you are reaching for can wait. If you think about it, very few things are so urgent they can't wait until morning.

- **Put the day to rest.** Resist the urge to engage with things related to your daily life. Do not indulge in thoughts of the day's events, tomorrow's to-do list, or work responsibilities. These things can wait until morning. Learn to shut them off and remove yourself from them after a specific time. If you struggle with this, try some distractions or say affirmations aloud to yourself, like "These things can wait; I deserve rest."

- **Do something that will help you relax physically.** Do things that encourage your body to release tension or de-stress. Try taking a warm bath, doing yoga or stretching, or even pausing for deep breaths. You can also try shimmying, wiggling, or shaking your body to release tension; do some humming; or try EFT tapping (also known as Emotional Freedom Technique tapping, a technique that involves tapping on specific pressure points, similar to acupressure).

- **Cuddle up to a pet or loved one.** Cuddling releases oxytocin, which is believed to reduce the impact of stress and mitigate cortisol. When you feel extra stressed, try reaching out to someone for a hug or snuggling up to your pet. Oxytocin is released in response to perceived social support, positive touch, and affirmative relationships. Even minor interactions can induce this effect, so reach out for some affection.

- **Look into getting a weighted blanket.** These blankets usually have small weights sewn into or attached to them and have been found to reduce anxiety and stress. Some studies even found that people sleeping with weighted blankets enjoyed an overall longer time asleep and moved around less while asleep.
- **Try herbal remedies.** There are quite a few herbal products that have been associated with improved sleep. They can also have a calming effect. Some examples are ashwagandha, passionflower, lemon balm, melatonin, magnesium, motherwort, and bacopa. As always, speak to a doctor before using these products.

USING THE RELAXATION RESPONSE TO MANAGE STRESS

Most of our biological functions are managed by the autonomic nervous system. One part of this system is the sympathetic nervous system that triggers the stress response. Another is the parasympathetic nervous system, which manages the relaxation response (also known as the rest-and-digest response).

This second one acts as an off-switch for fight-or-flight. It is what reverses the changes made by it once the initial threat has passed and is what returns normalcy to your body. When this response is activated, the heart slows, blood pressure decreases, and breathing evens. It also restaurants the systems that were paused by the stress reaction.

This response is usually activated automatically once the brain senses the stressor is gone. Still, this isn't always as effective in a world where the threat isn't as simple as a predator trying to eat you. The reality is that most of our stress is caused by things that do not simply go away. This means that the parasympathetic nervous system might not kick in when it should. On top of this, chronic stress makes the stress response hyperactive (i.e., easier to activate and harder to shut down). All of this combines to create an ineffective relaxation response.

However, since the relaxation response is a built-in feature of our brains, we can use it to our advantage to manage our stress. To do this, we must learn how to trigger it ourselves.

Benefits of using the relaxation response include

- less muscle tension
- better digestion and decreased gastrointestinal symptoms
- improved mood and better emotional regulation
- clearer thinking
- better-quality sleep
- increased resilience (how well you adapt to situations and manage unexpected circumstances)

HOW TO ENGAGE THE RELAXATION RESPONSE

In this section, I'll discuss a few methods through which you can trigger your relaxation response to decrease stress. Of course, these are not the only methods to do this, but they are some of the more effective and accessible ones.

Breathing Exercises

Breathing exercises are one of the most effective and convenient ways of triggering relaxation.

The vagus nerve is the main supporter of the parasympathetic nervous system. This nerve runs from the brain down into the chest and abdomen. Deep breathing stimulates it, which triggers the parasympathetic nervous system and relaxation response. This is a crucial stimulation since this nerve influences biological functions like heart rate, breathing, and digestion.

There are multiple breathing exercises you can try. I mentioned counted breathing in the previous chapter (where you time your breathing per a certain count), but another excellent breathing exercise is belly breathing or diaphragmatic breathing. If you're unfamiliar with this, it is a technique where you use your diaphragm to breathe instead of your chest. To try it out, follow these steps:

1. Lie on your back with one hand on your stomach and the other on your chest.
2. When you inhale, keep your chest still while letting your belly inflate with the breath. Use your hands as indicators for this. Focus on moving the hand on your stomach while keeping the other one still.
3. As you exhale, let your abdomen deflate.
4. Keep focusing on moving your stomach while you breathe.

Make sure to practice this regularly until you get the hang of it. It can be tricky if you've never done it before and it might take some deliberate effort before it becomes natural. This technique works well because it allows for deeper breathing using the diaphragm rather than the chest.

Meditation

Meditation targets both the body and the mind for stress relief. It lets you foster awareness of yourself and your environment while decreasing stress levels. There are various meditation practices, and most involve some form of stillness and awareness.

Dr. H. Benson, the doctor who first brought attention to the relaxation response, found that meditation can effectively trigger stress relief. He found that it's been used for this purpose for thousands of years and remains influential today. He further developed a meditation practice that aims to induce relaxation specifically.

This specific practice is known as autogenic relaxation, and it uses repetition and awareness to strengthen emotional control and regulation. To practice it, follow these steps:

1. Sit somewhere comfortable where you are separated from other people and distractions. Find a place where you feel safe and where you will be undisturbed. Make yourself comfortable.
2. Close your eyes and gradually slow your breathing.

3. While you sit there, find one word or sound to repeat. It's better to vocalize it and not just think about it. You can also use a mantra or prayer. Repeat that chosen thing and focus on it as you do so. If your thoughts stray, gently redirect yourself to the repetition. Do this for 10–20 minutes.

4. When you're ready, open your eyes. Don't jump up immediately to get back to the world. Coming out of meditation can be jarring, so take a moment to reacclimate and settle back into yourself. When you stand up, do so slowly.

For the best effect, this meditation needs to be practiced daily.

Progressive Muscle Relaxation

If you've researched self-care sleep strategies independently, you'll have come across this one. For progressive muscle relaxation, you tense and relax each muscle or area of the body individually while paying attention to it.

1. Find a place where you can lie or sit comfortably. Try to minimize disturbances and distractions, then close your eyes.

2. Begin at your head. Tense your forehead and scrunch your face up. Slowly increase the tension and hold it for a few seconds; then let those muscles relax.

3. Repeat the previous step as you move down your body. After your head, move to your shoulders and down your arms to your hands. Then, move on to your

abdomen, pelvis, and down your legs. Gradually increase the tension in each area before deliberately making the muscles relax. Move slowly.

This can take some getting used to. Most of us aren't used to targeting specific muscle groups like this. If it helps, use movement to encourage that tension. For example, clench your fist and flex your wrist if you're trying to tense your forearm.

If you are prone to muscle cramps, warm up your muscles before doing this exercise. If you have a musculoskeletal condition or an active injury, consult a doctor before you start.

Yoga, Tai Chi, or Qigong

These are ancient practices that involve meditative movement and breathing. They each work a little differently regarding their movement level, strength requirements, and how challenging they are. All three use dynamic movement to reduce tension and create a balance between the mind and body. As a side benefit, they will also count as regular exercise and can improve your physical strength and stability.

If you want to try this, ensure you are doing so safely. If you have any other health concerns, talk to a doctor before starting any of these. You also should not practice these while sleep-deprived or after taking a sleeping medication as both can affect your balance and lead to injury.

If these disciplines aren't for you, consider other forms of exercise like Pilates, barre, or strength training. Regular exercise has an immensely positive effect on stress and can even be an outlet for you to vent some frustration. On top of that, exercise can optimize your abilities, as well as lead to better health outcomes and improved sleep.

Body Scan

This technique is similar to progressive muscle relaxation in that you use it to bring awareness to specific areas of the body. Start at your feet and gradually work your way up. For each region, take time to notice the sensations there. In particular, notice where these parts connect, if they touch the floor, what temperatures they're at, or how they feel. Notice if they're comfortable, achy, tired, or tense. Don't try to change these areas; just spend time with each in order to notice them. Then, move on to the next area.

You can do this scan multiple times. Once you reach your head, reverse the process and repeat the scan, this time from the top down. The first scan is used to create an introduction. The second scan is used to notice if anything has changed or if your perception of these areas has changed.

This is a great way to spend some time in stillness, removed from stress and learn how to be with yourself. It can help you become more familiar with your body.

Visualization

With this technique, you use imagined imagery as a point of focus. You can imagine a picture, a place, or even an experience.

Don't limit yourself to visual expression. You can also add smells, sounds, and tastes. Pick imagery that makes you feel safe and relaxed. When done right, visualization can take you away from the stress you are experiencing to a place associated with relaxation. We might not be able to have a beach holiday at a whim, but we can imagine one whenever we need to.

For example, close your eyes and picture the ocean. Focus on the colors of the sand and the water. Imagine the motion of the waves ebbing and flowing. As each wave breaks, imagine the sounds that come with it. You can also time your breathing to the rhythm of the waves. As the tide pulls back, inhale. Exhale when the waves push outward and break onto the sand.

If you want to try this but need help, follow some guided visualizations.

4

HEALTHY HABITS FOR BETTER SLEEP

Small daily improvements are the key to staggering long-term results.

— UNKNOWN

When facing a problem, especially a health problem, we tend to focus on eliminating the causes. If the thing that causes sleep disturbances is gone, the disturbances will go with it, right? While that is correct, it isn't our only avenue of recourse.

With insomnia, we can take active steps to improve our sleep beyond eliminating the causes. This involves changing our sleep habits. These habits are collectively known as sleep hygiene. Good sleep hygiene means having habits that support a good night's sleep. This includes creating the right sleeping environment, managing your daily sleep schedule, and making specific dietary changes. Let's go through each of these habits one by one.

#1—YOUR SLEEP ENVIRONMENT

One of the quickest—and easiest—habits to manage is the sleep environment. Your sleep environment refers to the space in which you sleep, like your bedroom. Regardless of what that space is, it influences how you sleep.

Maintain the Purpose of the Sleep Environment

Simply put, your sleep environment should only be used for two things: sleep and sex. Activities like work, hobbies, eating, or even relaxing should all be done outside of it. This is so your brain will not learn to associate your bed with other activities.

If you can't isolate the room, try to isolate the bed. Do not sit and work in your bed if you can avoid it. Try to avoid turning your bedroom into a multipurpose space where possible. Since this is not always possible, consider ways to separate the space mentally. For example, have a separate lamp with a different colored light bulb that you switch on only when getting ready for bed.

Noise

The best sleep comes from a quiet environment. Even if you aren't waking up fully, noise can pull you out of deep sleep.

This is likely a vestige of a survival instinct to protect us from predators.

Ideally, your sleep environment should be relatively quiet. If you live in a city or near any busy road, you likely won't have too much control over this. If you can't eliminate all sounds, minimize them. Invest in a white noise machine to drown out external sounds. Most of our reactions come from sudden or new sounds in the environment or changes to it. If the noise is consistent, it won't have as much effect. Alternatively, try leaving a fan on or using some earplugs. You can even try adding soundproofing to your bedroom using sound-damp-ening curtains.

Light

Our built-in sleep-wake cycles are influenced by light. Bright light is associated with mornings and thus signals that it's time to wake up. Exposure to light triggers the release of cortisol, the hormone that triggers wakefulness. Once that light dims, the body produces melatonin, the hormone that induces relaxation and sleepiness. Research suggests that artificial lighting delays the production of melatonin. We are so surrounded by light that our brains don't quite get the memo to begin preparing for sleep.

As you get ready for sleep, dim the lighting in your room. At the same time, turn off all screens and devices. The blue light from them reads as natural light and influences melatonin produc-tion. Constant exposure to it during the evenings disrupts your internal regulation. For this reason, it's recommended that you take a break from screens starting around two hours before going to sleep.

This does not mean your room has to be pitch black during the night. Safety reasons could mean having some light in the room. If you rely on a nightlight for nighttime bathroom breaks, ensure it is low enough not to disturb your sleep. Consider moving it out into the hallway or the bathroom instead.

Temperature

Make sure your environment is at a comfortable temperature to support your sleep needs. If you like sleeping under blankets, make sure the room is cool enough so you won't overheat. If you get hot or cold quickly, make sure to account for this. Experts suggest an environmental temperature of roughly 60–70 degrees F (or 15–22 degrees C). However, this might not be ideal for everyone. Use your experiences as an indicator. If you wake up feeling too cold or hot, your room temperature isn't right.

If you cannot easily control the temperatures of your environment, try swapping out your bedding for something that's weather appropriate. You can also opt for different sleep clothes to mitigate any further issues.

Comfort

We all have different preferences for sleep comfort—some people like softer surfaces, others like theirs a bit firmer.

Whatever your preferences are, ensure you are comfortable in your bed of choice. Discomfort is a significant contributor to our sleep quality and having the right mattress and pillows can make a huge difference.

If your mattress is on the older side or you often wake up stiff and sore, it might be time for a new one. We all have different firmness preferences, but you'll also want to consider your weight and height when choosing one. If you share a bed and your partner has vastly different preferences, try to find a compromise where you both get what you want. Try adding some extra padding or a foam topper for some extra firmness.

Next comes pillows. This is also something that's largely up to personal preferences. Some people like firmer pillows, while others like softer ones. Consider their firmness and loft (how high they are). You can also take your sleeping position into account for pillows. People who sleep on their stomachs should use very thin pillows or go without them entirely. People who are primarily back sleepers should opt for something a little flatter, and side sleepers should go for something taller and firmer. It's all about finding pillows that support your head in the position you sleep in the most.

For better sleep comfort, things like sheets, blankets, and pillowcases can also be swapped. Go for textures you like against your skin and materials that correlate with your preferred temperatures. If you're easily hot, go for cotton or lighter materials. If you're easily cold, try more substantial sheets.

Tidiness and Cleanliness

Your sleep environment should be clean. Make sure to dust everywhere frequently to avoid any allergens and irritants. Wash your bedding often for the same reason.

Beyond that, the space should ideally be neat. Clutter and chaos in the environment make it harder to shut off. Clutter also gives you easy distractions. If your room is messy, try tidying things up and see if it makes a difference. Move everything unnecessary out of the bedroom if that's possible. Try and make it so you aren't using your bedroom as a storage space for odds and ends. If these items must be in the room, try to put them away and out of sight if possible. Once that's done, make a point of keeping it like that.

Pets, Partners, and Children

As much as we love the people and pets in our lives, sometimes they interfere with our sleep. Pets are the easiest to manage. If a pet is causing disruptions, ban them from the bedroom. I know they're cute and having them cuddle up to you is nice, but it's not worth sacrificing your sleep.

If you have kids, you know they can be unpredictable. You can do nothing about one of their occasional nightmares that result in disrupted sleep while you comfort your child. However, set some boundaries if your kids are keeping you awake beyond what's necessary. Your sleep is not worth less than theirs. Try instilling a rule that says they shouldn't come into your bedroom before a specific time unless it's an emergency.

Partners are a little more challenging to deal with since they tend to share our beds. We love sleeping next to our partners, right? The concept itself is lovely. In practice, though, this isn't always the case. If you're lucky, you and your partner have the same sleep schedule, habits, and preferences. If you're not, this lack of synchronicity might contribute to your insomnia. If they snore, they might have sleep apnea and should see a doctor. If there are incompatibilities, have a conversation to see if you can figure out a compromise. Maybe they're a night owl and they keep the lights on to read while you are trying to sleep. Maybe they move around a lot and you're a light sleeper. Regardless, take some time to try and find a solution. You can consider getting a more stable mattress to minimize moving, use earplugs and an eye mask, or establish a schedule where you respect each other's needs using quiet hours.

If these incompatibilities are extreme, consider sleeping in separate beds or rooms. This is commonly known as sleep divorce, but it is not nearly as bad as it might seem. For this, you and your partner can share a quiet, relaxing time before bed, but ultimately separate when it comes time to sleep.

Bathroom Visits

One of my least favorite things to do in the middle of the night is to get up to go to the bathroom. Luckily, there are ways to avoid this. Forgo any unnecessary drinking in the four or so hours before going to bed. You can also reduce caffeine during the latter half of the day. Caffeine is a diuretic and makes you urinate more often, which gives you another reason to avoid it after a certain point in the day. No matter what, go to the bathroom right before going to sleep.

If none of these things make a difference, see a doctor. Frequent nighttime urination can be a symptom of an underlying health concern.

#2—SET A SLEEP SCHEDULE

At its most basic, a proper sleep schedule means going to bed and getting up at the same time every day—even on weekends. However, with the unpredictability of our schedules, this can be difficult, especially if you're juggling more than just your own timetable.

But why, you might ask, is this so important? Does it really matter when I sleep if I'm getting enough hours?

Research has shown that those with a consistent sleep schedule experience better quality sleep. This is because it influences our internal clock (the circadian rhythm). The circadian rhythm determines many things about us, like when we get hungry. It also determines when certain hormones (like those responsible for managing the sleep-wake cycle) are produced. Maintaining a consistent sleep schedule supports this rhythm while an inconsistent one disrupts it.

Consistency also minimizes the chance of accumulating sleep debt. If you're constantly going to sleep at the same time and waking up when you need to, there's a smaller chance of finding yourself in situations when you aren't getting enough sleep.

The exact times of this schedule can vary from person to person. Sleep is managed by two cycles: sleep drive and the circadian rhythm. These things combine to determine how your body is regulating the sleep-wake cycle. In some people, this can mean feeling tired earlier in the day and rising naturally earlier in the mornings. For others, it can mean getting that second wind and not feeling tired until much later while feeling unrested early in the mornings. The ideal times for your sleep schedule will depend on you.

If you're unsure where you fall, Google "sleep chronotype quiz" and find the link on thesleepdoctor.com. Dr. M. Breus developed an entire quiz to consider your personality traits, sleeping habits, preferences, and more. Once you complete the quiz, Dr. Breus links you to a video containing more information on your personal chronotype. This can be extremely helpful in finding the right sleep schedule.

Regardless of this predisposition, maintaining a regular schedule, even if it doesn't align with your chronotype, will still have better effects than an irregular schedule.

The easiest way to pin down a sleep schedule is to ask yourself what time you need to be awake on average. You can then work backward from that time to figure out when you need to go to sleep. For example, if your work requires you to be awake at 7 a.m., your ideal bedtime (assuming you're an adult) is between 10 p.m. and midnight. If you stay up past then, you won't get enough sleep.

The Effects of an Irregular Sleep Schedule

We know already that sleep insufficiency has negative consequences, but how much does irregularity add to it? It isn't until much more recently that researchers have begun asking this question.

A 2020 study found a link between irregular sleeping patterns and the risk of developing heart disease (Huang et al., 2020). In this study, researchers measured nearly 2,000 participants' sleep habits and monitored them for five years. They found that the participants with irregular sleeping habits had more than double the risk of developing a heart-related complication than those with consistent sleep schedules. They concluded that irregular sleep patterns can be an independent risk factor for heart problems.

This same study also found a link between irregular schedules and metabolic disorders. They found that the participants with an irregular schedule had a higher rate of metabolic problems (like higher cholesterol, glucose levels, and larger waists). As mentioned above, this also contributed to their risk of developing heart disease. This persisted even after those participants adjusted their schedules to something more consistent. These participants were also showing more symptoms of depression, a higher likelihood of overeating, and more signs of sleep apnea.

Furthermore, irregular sleep schedules interfere with the natural functioning of the circadian rhythm. I briefly touched on this above, but to expand on this, the circadian rhythm acts as our internal clock. It determines the timing of many biological functions, including the sleep-wake cycle. When functioning correctly, this rhythm signals cortisol and melatonin production at the correct times. Irregular sleep schedules disrupt its functioning by suppressing the production of these hormones, particularly melatonin. Without it, our sleep becomes lighter and more fragmented. This means we have an overall more challenging time falling and staying asleep. This bleeds into other systems managed by the circadian rhythm like metabolism, the immune system, and the heart.

Our exposure to artificial light further complicates this circadian dysregulation. This is most predominantly seen in people who work night shifts. A recent study compared the sleep outcomes of day-shift workers and night-shift workers (Zhang et al., 2022). They found that those working night shifts had overall worse sleep quality and circadian rhythm activity. Initial results also showed that night-shift workers had less sleep duration, but that they could make up for the time differences through naps and longer sleep times while off-shift.

These irregularities have been found to persist for several years after the person begins regulating their sleep.

Another study found that people getting too little sleep and people on irregular schedules (i.e., sleeping in on the weekends) gained weight over a two-week period. Those same people also showed impaired insulin functionality compared to participants who maintained a regular schedule.

We already learned how bad it is not to get regular sleep, but now we also know how the regularity of our sleeping changes things. After more recent research, researchers concluded that your risk for these disadvantages multiplies for every hour of change in your sleep schedule. In the case of metabolic risks, like obesity and diabetes, these risks can multiply by as much as 27% (NHLBI, 2019).

Altogether, these studies concluded that irregular schedules contribute to the overall effect of sleep insufficiency. On top of this, catching up on sleep on the weekends might make up for overall time spent asleep, but it does not affect the overall outcomes of patients. Participants who technically got enough sleep but did so through an irregular schedule had the same adverse outcomes as those who weren't sleeping enough.

How to Fix Your Sleep Schedule and Reset Your Circadian Rhythm

1. Gradually reset your bedtime. Going to bed four hours earlier will be tough if you're used to being up until 2 a.m. Instead, slowly adjust your bedtime and wake time. A good recommendation is to scale it back 15 minutes at a time every two or three days. Be patient with yourself when you do this. Decide beforehand which days you will push back your schedule and then stick to it.

2. Don't take naps, even if it feels like you need one. I know it's hard, but trust me. Sleeping during the day will interfere with your sleeping at night. You're trying to reprogram your circadian rhythm, and napping will

interfere with that. Instead of napping, try light exercise when you feel tired or drowsy.

3. Manage your light exposure. Your circadian rhythm is influenced by light. When it registers brightness, it will signal the production of cortisol. For this reason, avoid light before bedtime. This doesn't have to mean existing in darkness until it's time to go to sleep. In the evenings, keep your surroundings dimmer. Avoid anything that gives off blue light like the TV, your phone, or the computer.

4. On the same note, use light to your advantage. Light indicates to your brain that it needs to be alert and awake. If your bedroom is fairly dark, open your curtains when you wake up. This exposure to natural light will set your circadian rhythm to start the day and help you stay on track to feel sleepy in the evening. You can also do this by spending time by a window or going outside.

5. Do not sleep in when you have the chance. Maintain your routine. Go to bed and wake up at the same time each day. Yes, even on weekends and vacations. Do not sleep in or lie around in bed—get up. Consistency is key in this process. Even one day off schedule can set you back some. Invest in a decent alarm clock and set a rule for yourself to never hit snooze.

6. Watch what you eat close to your bedtime. Avoid heavy foods that can cause heartburn or acid reflux. Steer clear of foods that have high sugar content. If you are hungry in the hours before sleep, go for something light and nutritious. Certain foods (like kiwis and cherries)

can even help you sleep better. A good rule of thumb is to stop eating around three hours before sleeping.

7. Exercise regularly. Frequent exercise can help regulate your circadian rhythm and biological functioning. You can even kill two birds with one stone and take a walk outside. That way, you get both your exercise and a good dose of natural light. That being said, don't exercise before bed. More activity during the day is generally known to help improve your sleep quality. However, exercise is stimulating. Working out too close to bedtime excites you and keeps you awake longer. If you want to squeeze in an evening workout, ensure you're done at least an hour before your chosen bedtime and cool down thoroughly afterward. Opt for lower-intensity exercises in that case.

8. Set the mood. Create a nighttime routine that will help you relax and get ready for sleep. Fill the hour or so before sleep with a consistent schedule of relaxing activities. Choose things that will help you relax and unwind. For example, a warm bath, listening to some music, a destressing meditation, or reading. These things will help you de-escalate and warm you up for sleep. Performing them in the same order and at the same times each night will also teach your body to associate them with sleep.

9. If nothing works and you cannot get your sleep schedule fixed, no matter what you try, schedule a visit with your doctor. It could be that there is some underlying issue that's interfering with your scheduling attempts. Your doctor will also be able to guide you

more specifically on things you can do during the process.

Keep in mind that this can take some time. How long it will take depends on your circumstances, how long you've been experiencing irregular sleep and your sleep needs. It takes time to get to the point where the new schedule sets in and then even more time to adjust to this new schedule.

Don't get upset at yourself if it doesn't work out on the first try, either. Remember, you are reprogramming an automatic function, which takes time and discipline. If it feels like it isn't working, give it time. It's generally recommended to wait a month or two after settling on the new schedule before making any decisions. Once you have worked up to that new schedule, give it time to settle in before you decide whether it's working. In the meantime, stick with it. This takes discipline. Again, even one day off schedule can set you back.

#3—QUIT CAFFEINE BY NOON

Caffeine is a plant-based, organic stimulant commonly used to combat drowsiness. It is reasonably fast-acting and peaks around 30–60 minutes after consumption. Caffeine stays in your system longer than you might think, with a 3–5 hour half-life. Half-life measures how long it takes a person's body to process half of a particular substance. This means that the effects of caffeine can still be seen more than five hours after consuming it.

This has both positive and negative effects. On the one hand, caffeine endorses alertness. It's been known to influence mood, mental clarity, reaction times, and mental performance. On the other hand, it impacts our sleep. It affects our circadian rhythm and even reduces the amount of deep sleep we get.

Caffeine is an adenosine receptor antagonist. This means it blocks receptors from binding to adenosine. What's adenosine now? Adenosine is a hormone that is produced throughout the day and promotes sleepiness. It builds up while you're awake and makes you feel gradually more tired as the day progresses. Having this process blocked is detrimental to your quality of sleep.

Worst of all, your body can develop a natural tolerance to caffeine. The more of it you drink, the more you'll need for the same effect. Eventually, you'll find yourself in a position where you consume more than the recommended amount to make up for the sleep you aren't getting.

Like everything else, caffeine has its benefits and drawbacks. While it has not been shown to be a direct cause of insomnia, it still contributes to it. In other words, caffeine aggravates its symptoms and worsens the problem, especially since we rely on it when we don't sleep well. Luckily, this does not mean you have to quit your caffeinated drink of choice; it only means limiting when you drink it.

When to Stop Drinking Caffeine

This can vary from person to person. There is no ideal cut-off time. What time you should stop drinking caffeine will depend on several factors, like

- the typical amount of caffeine you consume per day
- how well you metabolize it
- the caffeine content of your preferred drink
- your predisposition toward sleep disturbances

The average recommended cut-off point is around 6 hours before your planned bedtime. If you want to sleep at 10 p.m., the cut-off is around 2 p.m. However, if you still find that you're having difficulty falling asleep or staying asleep, it's worth cutting off caffeine earlier to see if that will make a difference.

Note here that this isn't limited to coffee. Caffeine is found in many drinks and even some foods. Coffee, certain teas, and energy drinks have the highest amounts of caffeine, but you should also check the ingredients in your medications. If you are taking medication that contains some, speak to your doctor about changing when you take it or ask about alternatives.

#4—MIND WHAT YOU EAT BEFORE BED

The food we eat, when we eat it, and our food choices influence our sleeping patterns. Furthermore, our sleep quality also affects our food choices. To recap, those who sleep poorly are prone to poorer dietary choices. Poor sleep slows their metabolism and influences the hormones that indicate when they feel full. This results in overeating and relying on food to compensate for lost energy.

What we haven't explored a great deal yet is how our diet influences our sleep. Eating before bed is generally bad, but it goes beyond that. Your circadian rhythm determines when you get hungry. If you make sudden changes to your diet or change when you eat, that rhythm is thrown off and so is sleep.

Your body works a lot like a general corporation. At the head of everything is the circadian rhythm. It makes executive decisions and tells the other departments when to do certain things. If one of those departments changes its schedule, the circadian rhythm must adjust to that change. Everything needs to coordinate for the body to function effectively and having one system out of whack will affect everything else.

So, how do you put this into practice for sleep? The best thing you can do is maintain a healthy, balanced diet and avoid certain food before bedtime. Research has shown that people with diets low in fiber but high in saturated fats and sugars experience poorer quality sleep. The recommendations are to eat nutritious food, avoid processed sugars and saturated fats, and eat healthy portions.

This is especially important for people who experience sleep difficulties. Poor sleep leads to metabolic issues. It also leads to overeating, higher risks of diabetes and metabolic issues, and poor decision-making. This means our diets get poorer when we aren't sleeping well. Your diet might have been affected without you even knowing, so it's important to make the deliberate decision to eat better for your sleep and well-being.

When to Stop Eating

There are a few reasons why eating right before bed can be a bad idea. One is that the metabolic process is slowed down by sleep. Every time you eat, your body must process the food, move it through the digestive tract, and absorb nutrients. This takes active work and takes a bit longer than you'd expect. If you eat before sleeping, this process could still be active while your body is trying to slow down. Furthermore, lying down means your body must work harder to move the food to the intestines. Because of this, eating before bed causes things like heartburn and stomach aches.

Another reason to avoid it is that late-night eating leads to overeating. Some studies have shown that nighttime eating is less filling than daytime eating, meaning it takes longer to feel full.

Most experts recommend stopping around 2–3 hours before bedtime to avoid these things. If you have a slower metabolism, this time might need to be longer. These guidelines are only recommendations and are by no means hard rules. There are medical circumstances that might require eating before going to bed. If you have a health condition impacted by food, talk to a doctor before changing your diet. Your culture and religion might also influence when you eat. You must decide what is good for you, and if there are situations in your life that mean you have to eat late at night, then do so.

What If You're Hungry Before Bed?

Depending on your chosen bedtime, you might be juggling sleep and dinner. If that is the case, do not skip dinner solely for the sake of sleep. In this case, I am talking about snacking before bed.

Hunger is a basic physical need and usually indicates that it's either time to eat per your circadian rhythm or that you need food. Sometimes, ignoring this hunger right before bed is the best choice, but not always. Below are a few scenarios where it is okay to go to bed without eating if you're hungry and situations where it is not okay.

Going to bed hungry is okay if

- you are making changes to your eating habits in pursuit of a healthier lifestyle and still adjusting to the new routine
- you are cutting calories for health reasons or when following an intermittent fasting diet (only if you are still getting enough calories and nutrients throughout the rest of the day, though)
- you're hungry because of lack of sleep
- you often experience acid reflux or heartburn during the night

It is not okay to go to sleep without eating if

- you are undernourished or are not meeting nutritional standards
- you are not eating regularly or missed a meal during the day
- you are prone to or at risk of having low blood sugar
- you have type 1 diabetes
- you are trying to build muscles or have an intense workout regime that requires muscle repair
- your hunger is so intense that it will disrupt your sleep

There are pros and cons when it comes to going to bed hungry. On the one hand, you avoid the symptoms and complications of sleeping on a full stomach. On the other hand, hunger can keep you awake and limit your body's ability to repair and regenerate tissue. If you are concerned about this, or want better insight, speak to a healthcare provider. If you have any health condition related to food in any way, speak to a doctor before making a decision.

The key to mastering this is distinguishing between feeling hungry and peckish. Are you hungry or do you just feel like eating? If you need to eat, look at the next section to see which foods to avoid and which foods are good options for pre-bedtime eating.

Healthy Bedtime Snacks Versus Foods to Avoid

Some foods are better than others for late-night eating. Certain foods aggravate insomnia symptoms or contribute to the processes that keep you awake, while others can promote healthy sleep.

Healthy food choices are:

- **Almonds:** Almonds are highly nutritious and are believed to help prevent diabetes and heart disease. They contain a good amount of magnesium, which has been shown to affect sleep positively. Their main benefit comes from them being a source of melatonin, the sleep hormone.
- **Turkey:** This meat is a fantastic source of protein and other nutrients. Protein has been shown to improve sleep, with many believing it helps promote deeper sleep. Turkey also contains tryptophan, a chemical that boosts melatonin production.
- **Kiwi:** Kiwis contain vitamins C and K, fiber, antioxidants, folate, and potassium. This gives them high nutritional value. One study found that people who ate one or two kiwis before bed fell asleep roughly 40% easier (Lin et al., 2011). These participants also slept longer and fell asleep easier. It's believed that this is because kiwis are a natural source of serotonin (a hormone that regulates the transition between sleep and wakefulness).

- **Tart cherries and tart cherry juice:** This one is particularly well-known for its effects on insomnia. Tart cherries contain magnesium, phosphorus, potassium, and melatonin. Several studies found that tart cherry juice leads to longer sleep time and better sleep quality.
- **Fatty fish:** Fatty fish (like salmon, trout, and mackerel) are good sources of vitamin D and omega-3 fatty acids. Both have key roles in the production of serotonin. This makes it a good source of protein for meals and a good option for a bedtime snack.
- **Walnuts:** Walnuts have an excellent reputation as a healthy food source. Not only do they contain various vitamins and minerals, but they are also a source of omega-3 fatty acids. On top of this, walnuts are one of the best sources of melatonin.
- **Chamomile tea:** While not necessarily a food, I include this one since you cannot have a list of sleep-promoting dietary options without chamomile. Chamomile contains flavones that reduce inflammation in the body. It also contains apigenin, a chemical that binds to your neuroreceptors to promote sleepiness. It's been found to relieve insomnia and depression symptoms. Studies have shown that people who regularly drink chamomile tea fall asleep easier, stay asleep longer, and experience better quality rest.
- **Passionflower tea:** Passionflower is another herb that is believed to promote sleep. Like chamomile, it is a source of apigenin. It is also thought that it supports the production of GABA, which is essential in managing

chemicals that promote stress. As such, passionflower can be a good way to calm down and relax before bed.

Other good foods for sleep include milk, bananas, oatmeal, yogurt, and unsalted nuts and seeds. These foods are not as well studied for their effects on sleep but can help due to their nutritional value.

Foods to avoid at night:

- **Heavy foods and large meals:** Some foods are easier to digest than others. Some foods also cause more discomfort than others. With that in mind, avoid foods that make you feel full and heavy. For example, burgers, steaks, or fries. This also includes most fast foods. Related to this, avoid big meals right before bedtime. Sleeping with a full stomach can be uncomfortable regardless of how healthy the food is. If a food gives you that "too full to move" feeling, it's not acceptable as a bedtime snack.
- **Foods with a high-water content:** Most foods, especially plant-based ones, have some water in them. This can vary. Fluids from food are still processed the same way as fluids from drinks. Eating foods with a high-water content can lead to more trips to the bathroom. Examples of these foods are celery, watermelon, and cucumber.
- **Foods with hidden caffeine:** Some foods can have small doses of caffeine in them. Even decaf coffee still has traces of caffeine. Check nutritional labels before

choosing something as a late-night meal. Look for chocolates, sodas, teas, and anything coffee flavored.

- **Sugary treats and food with a high glucose index (GI) value:** Foods with a high sugar content cause fluctuations in blood sugar levels. Low blood sugar has been found to disrupt sleep, while high blood sugar has been found to make a person feel sleepy. However, changes in your blood sugar level can trigger the release of various hormones to reduce it. Once it has dropped, the change can disrupt the rest of your sleep. Foods to avoid because of this include processed sweets, white bread, foods high in carbs, and anything to which you add sugar.

- **Tyramine-rich foods:** Tyramine is an amino acid that promotes brain activity. For this reason, it is recommended to avoid foods that contain it toward the end of the day. For example, tomatoes, red wine, and soy sauce. These foods are not necessarily bad; you just shouldn't eat them as a late-night snack.

- **Spicy foods:** Spicy foods tend to cause heartburn. At the same time, they raise your body temperature. That feeling you get from being hot after eating something spicy can cause you to struggle when falling asleep. Again, this does not mean you have to cut out all spicy foods; you just have to eat them a little earlier in the day.

- **Acidic foods:** Like spicy foods, acidic foods can trigger heartburn and gastrointestinal discomfort. Avoid anything with high acidic content. This does not mean just avoiding anything sour. Foods in this category include most condiments (especially tomato sauce), white wine, raw onions, and anything citrusy.

- **Foods that make you gassy:** Gas is a natural byproduct of human digestion. Foods that are heavy in fiber can lead to a build-up of gas in the intestines. If you're lying down, the pressure in them changes. This might aggravate the feeling of gas build-up and cause discomfort. No one likes feeling bloated, and that's precisely what this can lead to. Avoid dried fruits, high-fiber fruits and vegetables, and beans close to bedtime. These things are fantastic for your nutrition but not necessarily for your sleep.

#5—LIMIT ALCOHOL

While alcohol can help you fall asleep, it does not improve the quality of your rest, quite the opposite. Alcohol is a nervous system depressant. This means it suppresses brain activity and will make you sleepy and relaxed. Many people find that it helps them fall asleep, and research reflects this. Despite this, though, alcohol has other effects that far outweigh this minor benefit.

First of all, it's essential to recognize that your body can build up a tolerance for alcohol. You get desensitized to its sedative effects and will eventually need to start drinking more to get it. One or two glasses already come with adverse effects; increasing the amount of alcohol will only make them worse.

Alcohol is known to decrease REM sleep. REM sleep is an important part of the cycle since this is where most cognitive and emotional restoration occurs. When this is reduced, the person will experience more mood disturbances and stress, which might prompt them to sleep worse and drink more.

Directly after taking a drink, your body will start to metabolize the alcohol. This is a lengthy process; while the alcohol remains in your system, your nervous system is depressed. This makes it easier to fall asleep and can even result in deeper stage 3 sleep while it is still in your system. However, once that alcohol is processed, the body experiences a rebound effect that leads to spikes in brain activity. As a result, the latter half of the night is characterized by lighter sleep, frequent waking, and mental arousal.

Alcohol is a diuretic—it makes you urinate more. Drinking in the evening can lead to more frequent trips to the bathroom. The bladder is usually more inactive during the night, and having it be more active—by, say, filling it up with alcohol— disrupts sleep.

Additionally, research has shown that moderate drinking within an hour of sleep disrupts melatonin production, making it harder to fall asleep and causing irregularities in the sleep- wake cycle. This then affects the circadian rhythm for the next day, leading to sleep disruption the next night.

In summary, drinking leads to fragmented sleep, less REM sleep, and irregular sleep-wake cycles. Even moderate drinking can lead to these effects, but the more you drink, the worse this gets.

How Much Drinking Is Okay?

Research suggests that even one drink at the wrong time can lead to adverse sleep effects, regardless of personal tolerance. According to the Sleep Foundation (Pacheco, 2020), low amounts of alcohol can decrease your sleep by more than 9%, moderate amounts by 24%, and high amounts by 39%. In this context, moderate drinking equals one drink for women and two for men.

It's generally recommended to wait four to six hours between drinking and sleep. While the body can process alcohol in an hour, studies have found that melatonin is repressed up to three hours after stopping. One study even found residual effects of alcohol on sleep up to six hours later.

This recommendation is based on the average person's response to alcohol. Your best cut-off point will depend on your circumstances and factors like age, sex, physical fitness, how much you drink, and how often you consume alcohol. The more you drink at one time, the longer you will have to wait. Please note, however, that this does not mean pushing off sleep based on your drinking. Alcohol is not an excuse to stay up late. These are guidelines for determining when to stop drinking based on your chosen bedtime.

Best Drinking Practices

If you want to drink while promoting the best sleep possible, use the following tips for the best drinking practices.

- Wait at least three hours between drinking and sleeping. If you want to sleep at eleven, that means no more drinks after eight.
- Drink plenty of water to rehydrate and help your body process the alcohol.
- Eat alongside your drink or drink alongside your meals. This can help your body manage the alcohol while also helping you limit your drinking. If you drink at regular mealtimes, for example, it can help you know when to stop and keep your drinking to a suitable schedule.
- Do not drink if you are taking sleeping medications. Alcohol and sleeping pills are both nervous system depressants. Using both means more suppression than is recommended. This can lead to suppressed breathing, a higher risk of injury, or issues with swallowing and choking.

How to Sober Up for Sleep

This section contains tips for reducing alcohol intake to ensure it does not affect your sleep. If you find that you cannot stop or cut back despite how it affects your sleep, you might have a drinking problem. Reach out to a healthcare provider for advice on how to better manage this.

Now, there's not a lot you can do to speed up how fast your body processes alcohol. You can't force yourself to sober up quicker. However, you can take steps to reduce the effect of alcohol on your sleep should you find yourself drinking later in the evening than planned. In other words, you can take steps to reduce how it influences your sleep tomorrow. These steps can also help you be more mindful of your drinking.

1. Create healthier coping mechanisms or develop other ways of destressing. We need time to destress and wind down because of how complicated life is and how much stress affects our health. For many people, alcohol is a way to do that. It's a fairly effective means of relaxing despite not being a healthy coping mechanism. Instead of relying on a drink or two to relax, try to find something else to wind down. Try listening to an audiobook, doing light stretching, or picking up a calming hobby. You can also use journaling before bed to process the day's events.

2. Stop drinking early enough. Use the recommended four to six hours to determine when to stop drinking. If you still find your sleep fragmented, try stopping earlier to see if that will help. Adjust your routine to find a time frame that works for you.

3. Create a drinking plan and set a limit. Take a moment to develop a drinking plan that clearly sets out when and how much you drink on those occasions. Once you have it, stick to it. If you have a limit on the number of drinks you allow yourself, make sure to keep track of your drinks as you go. The same is true for time. If you're scheduled to stop at a certain time, keep an eye on the clock to ensure you stick to the limit. You can even set an alarm to warn you when it's time to stop.

4. See a doctor if you rely on alcohol as a sleeping aid and talk to them about healthier alternatives.

5. Substitute drinks for nonalcoholic or low-alcohol drinks. Instead of going for your regular drink of choice, try something that has lower alcohol levels—or perhaps none at all. Plenty of drinks will give you the same taste or satisfy the habit with fewer adverse effects. If you're used to drinking a glass of wine with dinner and want to keep up the habit, try replacing it with a glass of juice or consider diluting it with ice or water. While any amount of alcohol can have adverse effects, weaker alcohol will affect you less severely.

6. Get a good bottle stopper. If you're a big wine drinker, you'll know that once you've opened a bottle, it doesn't keep. Instead of finishing off an entire bottle to keep it from being wasted, use a bottle stopper to extend its shelf life.

7. Familiarize yourself with standard serving sizes. The recommendations for drinking practices are based on standard serving sizes. This varies from drink to drink based on alcohol content. A standard serving of whiskey looks very different from one of wine. Learn what qualifies as a standard serving of your drink of choice, then pay attention to your consumption. Limit yourself to a certain number of servings (ideally around one or two).

8. Understand your drinking triggers and avoid them. Certain situations are more suitable for drinking than others, and we tend to drink more in those situations. Drinking triggers can also be events, people, or circumstances. Once you've identified your triggers, try to find ways to minimize your exposure to them to

avoid drinking more than you'd like. For example, if you know you drink more when stressed, avoid going to places like bars or buying alcohol when you know you're stressed.

9. Stay accountable. Drinking is a habit that's difficult to shake. It's addictive for a reason. As such, drinking less is not always as simple as deciding to cut back. Find someone you trust and talk to them about your plans. Explain to them why you want to cut back and keep them up to date on your progress. Sharing these things with others makes them more real and can be a great motivator to stay on track. Part of being accountable is being honest about your intentions and progress.

10. Spend time with people who respect your boundaries and desire to cut back. Drinking is something we tend to do in social situations, and as such, socializing can often be a place where we drink more than we want to. If you're trying to cut back and your friends are being pushy, they might not be the right company for you while you do this. Instead, surround yourself with people who would respect your choices and not try to push you into breaking them.

If you drink more than planned or much later than anticipated, do not let it influence your sleep schedule. It's better to go to bed at the regular time and sleep poorly for one night than it is to wait up and lose progress. Yes, your sleep won't be great, but it won't affect your overall progress as much as delaying sleep would. Instead, do some things that can minimize your struggle during the night and the following day. Drink plenty of water and keep an extra glass and some painkillers on hand for the next morning. Forego any sleeping medication you might usually take.

If you drank heavily, it is not safe to go to bed. In that case, you should stay up until the alcohol has left your system. Going to sleep while heavily intoxicated can have potentially dangerous consequences, like choking on vomit.

IN SUMMARY

The way you approach your daily life impacts how you sleep. With some dedication and discipline, you can make the necessary changes in your routine to improve your sleep. These lifestyle changes will often do more for you than any sleeping pill ever will.

To summarize, for the best possible sleep, you need an appropriate sleep environment that is clean and neat, an effective sleep schedule, and the right diet. You should avoid light and noise disturbances during the night, cut off caffeine and alcohol early enough, and put away technology to avoid disrupting your circadian rhythm and losing sleep.

UNRAVEL THE MYSTERY OF GREAT SLEEP AND HELP OTHERS ACHIEVE THEIR DAILY GOALS WITH ENERGY AND VITALITY

"The reasons we can't sleep at night are usually the same reasons we don't truly live during the day."

— MICHAEL XAVIER

In the introduction, I highlighted the vital link between sleep and mental health. It is incredibly difficult to weather life's challenges with grace, calm, and a positive mindset, when you are exhausted and fatigued, and every cell in your body is screaming for rest.

Despite the importance of good rest, the prevalence of sleep disorders means that when someone tells you they are struggling to fall asleep, or they have had a four-hour night of sleep, it almost seems typical. Finding people who have aced the science and art of good sleep is increasingly difficult and as a society, we have come to accept sleep deprivation as just another part of modern, stressful life.

Very few people know that insomnia is usually completely manageable. Nor are they aware of the vital links between the choices they make and the sleep they get. Many are surprised to discover that their sleep environment matters greatly to the quickness with which they fall asleep—and stay asleep!

By now, you have discovered so many strategies that invite you to take a whole new viewpoint when it comes to sleep quantity and quality. You know that a good rest starts with your mindset and that tackling stress proactively is vital if you want to avoid running through problems at night. You have also honed a host of relaxation exercises that can help you bring your mind back to the present moment and release built-up tension.

By leaving a review of this book on Amazon, you'll show other readers that they're not the only ones facing sleeping challenges, and you'll reveal where they can find exactly what they need to eliminate the root causes of poor sleep.

Simply by letting other readers know how this book has helped you and what they can expect to find inside, you'll provide vital knowledge to someone else – and help them get rid of the bad habits that are stopping them from feeling energized in the morning.

Thank you so much for your support. Helping others enjoy a good night's sleep can have a profound effect on your personal and professional life. The more rest people get, the more likely they are to energetically go for their goals... and the butterfly effect of this mindset is tremendous.

5

EXERCISING FOR BETTER SLEEP

> *Get a daily workout, and you will naturally eat and sleep better. You will be a different person. Exercise will enhance your performance in your daily hours.*

— JOHN SOFORIC

EFFECT OF REGULAR EXERCISE ON SLEEP

It's common knowledge that exercise is good for us, but does this extend to sleep? A 2012 critical review of studies analyzed the results of multiple studies to see whether exercise was a viable treatment tool for insomnia. Across the board, they found exercise as effective as sleeping pills (Passos et al., 2012). Furthermore, a 2015 review found that while regular exercise was overall more beneficial, even a single workout resulted in better sleep (Kredlow et al., 2015).

In many ways, sleep and physical activity are mutually beneficial systems. The more active you are, the better you sleep, and
vice versa. This is due to a few reasons.

Firstly, exercise increases adenosine. If you recall, adenosine is
a hormone that builds up in your brain the longer you are
awake. The more of it you have at the end of the day, the better
you sleep. Regular exercise increases your natural adenosine
levels and thus supports the sleep-wake cycle.

Secondly, regular exercise promotes good sleep quality. More
active people spend more time in stage 3 and stage 4 sleep. This
means they get more rest and benefit from longer periods of
restoration. Why exercise does this is still largely unclear, but
some experts believe it might be because exercise triggers
earlier release of melatonin.

Thirdly, exercise improves your mental health. It does so
primarily by triggering the release of feel-good hormones. This
makes you less reactive to stress, induces relaxation, and
improves your mood. It's also been proven to help manage
symptoms of depression and anxiety and lessen stress. This
means that it not only improves your sleep on a biological level
but also addresses some of the psychological influences that
cause insomnia.

Fourth, regular exercise is an outlet for pent-up energy.
Modern life only requires a little physical movement. Many of
us spend hours sitting down without any reason to move
around. In short, we become sedentary. This often means we
don't expend all the energy we have stored up. Increasing your
physical activity helps tip the scale in favor of sleep. It makes

you more tired, thus making it easier to doze off at night. It also counteracts the adverse effects of inactivity and promotes a healthier lifestyle.

Lastly, exercise minimizes the symptoms and effects of sleep apnea and chronic conditions that cause insomnia. It's been known to lessen pain, improve digestion, strengthen the heart, and optimize functionality.

WORKOUTS FOR GOOD SLEEP

We know that exercise helps you sleep, but does that extend to all kinds of exercise, or are there specific types of activity that have better results?

Most studies and reviews focus on aerobic exercises. Aerobics (more commonly known as cardio) is an umbrella term that describes physical activities that get you moving for extended periods of time. These exercises are usually based on endurance and make use of repetitive movements to increase your heart rate and breathing. Types of aerobics are distinguished based on their level of intensity.

Moderate-intensity aerobics include walking, water exercising, and low-intensity cycling. With this kind of exercise, you could still maintain a conversation.

High-intensity aerobics are exercises that really push your heart rate and endurance. They include running, dancing, swimming, and active sports like basketball or volleyball. When doing these exercises, you would typically be able to speak up to a few words without running out of breath.

Most research on the effect of exercise on sleep is done using moderate-intensity aerobics. A few studies used different kinds of activities with the same results, which supports the idea that other forms of exercise would be just as beneficial.

Aside from aerobics, the following can also be used to improve your sleep:

- **Resistance training:** An anaerobic exercise using external force like weight or resistance to build muscles and strength. Resistance training exercises include body-weight workouts (like push-ups and sit-ups), weightlifting, and Pilates. Like aerobics, resistance workouts have been known to improve depression and anxiety symptoms, improve health outcomes, and increase sleep time.
- **Yoga:** A specific type of resistance training that uses meditative practices, breathing techniques, and postures (or poses). As a discipline, it decreases stress, builds strength, and improves health outcomes. While yoga has not been as exhaustively studied as other disciplines for sleep specifically, it has been found to work well with specific demographics (namely, the elderly and women with sleep problems and diabetes). This does not mean it is ineffective for other groups, just that it has not been studied in those groups to the same degree. However, yoga is a well-studied practice proven to decrease stress and improve health in all demographic groups. If yoga isn't your scene, but you want something similar, consider tai chi or qigong.

They use similar practices but are less physically demanding.

- **Walking:** Walking might not be the quickest way to get fit, but it is one of the best exercises for sleep. Walking is relaxing. It allows you to clear your head and relax. If you do it outside during the day, it also exposes you to natural light. It has all the benefits of other exercises without the physical strain of the more intense workout options. Walking can be a good starting point for those who are not habitual exercisers, and it is a safe alternative for those with medical conditions that make exercise difficult. Ideally, take a 20–30-minute walk outside in the late afternoon or early evening. Set a pace that feels comfortable. You can listen to music or put on a podcast to help you unwind. You can also do this with a friend for some company. While a deliberate walk is more beneficial, you can manage by increasing your average daily step count. If you want to walk but don't have a safe space to do it in, try walking in place at home.
- **Jumping rope:** Few people think about jumping rope when looking for exercises to help them sleep. However, it's a repetitive action that requires physical exertion. Counting each repetition can give your mind something to do instead of thinking and be a great way to unwind. Make sure to go at your own pace and remember that jumping is a high-impact activity.
- **Running:** Running or jogging is a higher-intensity aerobic exercise. It's a more intense version of walking that you can do anywhere. Running gives you an outlet

for your energy and is an effective way to destress. The bonus here is that you can do it outside to reap the benefits of extra natural light. Again, you can do this while listening to music or a podcast or with a friend.

- **Flexibility training:** These are exercises that target your mobility and agility. They are great for counteracting stiffness or targeting aching muscles. This usually takes the form of static or dynamic stretching, both good means of relaxation. Since they are less active, they can be used closer to bedtime to help you unwind. Stretching is also an excellent addition to any other workout for warming up and cooling down afterward.

IT'S ALL ABOUT TIMING

While research has repeatedly shown how exercise benefits sleep, there's little research on how timing affects it. For a long time, experts believed that nighttime exercising would be detrimental to sleep, but newer research suggests the opposite.

There is no one perfect time for exercising. The timing that works for you will depend on your schedule, sleep chronotype, health circumstances, and personal preferences. Most people would not experience adverse effects from moderate-intensity exercise in the evenings, provided they allow themselves time to cool off before sleeping.

Exercise triggers the release of certain hormones that lead to mental arousal and hyperactivity. Many people have an elevated mood after a good workout, which can stop them from winding down for sleep. On that note, you should give your body enough time to even out these hormones before trying to go to bed.

Furthermore, exercise increases your body temperature, which directly contradicts what the body naturally does for sleep. Fortunately, the body cools down around 60–90 minutes after working out. This mimics what happens when you sleep, so timing this right can encourage sleep. The general recommendation is to finish exercising at least one to two hours before trying to go to sleep.

Some research suggests that this can be different for morning people. While exercising before bed does not adversely affect night owls, early risers might find it disrupts their sleep. The best bet is to exercise at a time that feels good for you. That might be in the morning, during the day, or in the evenings.

As a rule, keep higher intensity exercises earlier in the day and less strenuous ones for the evening. A walk or stretching is unlikely to impact your sleep, while a vigorous run right before bed might—experiment with what works best for you.

CREATE A FITNESS PLAN

A fitness plan is one way to manage all the ins and outs of regular exercise. If you're just getting started, exercising can be intimidating. It's hard to know where to start, what to work on today, or how much of each exercise you should do. If you're not used to it, it becomes overwhelming quickly.

Like everything else, exercise is easier when it is part of a routine and planned in advance. A fitness plan does exactly that —it schedules your workouts and defines the details of your routines. This plan will include the type of exercises for each day, how many of them you should do, and how long you should do them. Think of it as a kind of recipe for your workouts.

Fitness plans make it easier to stay on track, meet your goals, and stick to a routine. A workout plan also

- ensures consistency in your workouts
- prevents over- and under-training
- ensures a balance between types of exercises
- provides a solid structure to follow
- works goals into the plan
- prevents burnout by including variety and removing uncertainty
- eliminates excuses like "Oh, I'll just do it tomorrow," or "I don't have time today"

Thorough fitness plans can also include nutritional plans and sleep schedules. Altogether, it ensures you get the most benefits out of your workouts as possible. It also removes a lot of the uncertainty and indecision. With a fitness plan, you don't have to figure out what you will do today; you can do what's on the plan without worrying about what you did last time or what you'll do next time.

How to Make a Fitness Plan

You can approach a personal trainer or workout coach to create a fitness plan or make one yourself. If you make one yourself, consider the following things:

- **What is your current level of fitness?** Before you can start anything, you need to know your current capabilities. Take the time to create a baseline. Record your weight, measurements, resting heart rate, how long it takes you to walk a certain distance (or how many steps you can do in six minutes), and how many squats, push-ups, and sit-ups you can do in 30 seconds. This will give you a good idea of where you're at and will also give you stats to recheck for a progress update. Regularly reevaluate your fitness level to ensure your plan stays up-to-date and effective.
- **What are your goals?** Create a few achievable but challenging goals for yourself. Make them as specific as possible. Avoid vague goals like "I want to lose weight," or "I want to sleep better." Your goals should be measurable and set to a specific timeline. For example, "I want to lose 15 pounds in two weeks," or "I want to be able to do 1,000 steps in 6 minutes."
- **Pick activities you like when choosing exercises and find alternatives for the ones you don't.** The more you dislike an activity, the less likely you are to keep up with it. If you hate running, don't include it in your fitness program. Instead, find something that works the same muscle groups and has the same effect. In other

words, find a suitable high-intensity aerobic exercise that will work your muscles, test your endurance, and increase your heart rate, like swimming or cycling. If you can't find an alternative, consider ways to make the exercise more fun.

- **Plan for progression.** The stronger you get, the more capable you'll become. If you're starting out, plan for a slow start. However, include an increase in difficulty in your plan. You will eventually get more robust, and your exercise habits should change to match that. If your workouts stay the same, your progress will stagnate.

- **Make space for exercise in your routine.** Schedule time to exercise in your daily life like you would a doctor's appointment or meeting. Don't leave it up to chance or figure you'll do it when you have time. Plan for it. This will help you keep up with it and ensure you stay consistent.

- **Don't repeat the same workout every time.** Instead, plan for variety. Include different kinds of exercises into your schedule. Aim to have at least one aerobic, strength training, and flexibility session per week. You can add a little bit of everything into your daily schedule, but it also helps to spread things out, so you aren't doing the same thing every day.

- **Allow enough time for rest and repair in between workouts.** Make sure you include rest days and enough time between sessions to ensure you aren't overdoing it. Allow at least 24–48 hours between workouts that use the same muscle groups. You can add other types of exercise in between. For example, if you do a leg routine on Monday, don't do other leg-intensive exercises the next day. Instead, try a moderate-intensity cardio workout or some yoga before returning to leg exercises. Alternatively, you can shift to another area of the body for the next day. For example, focus on the arms or core after a leg workout.

Write your fitness plan down. Don't just make plans in your head and leave it at that. Put it on paper—make it firm. This removes the chance for mix-ups and minimizes possible confusion.

Once you have a plan, find the right space. You can go to a gym, but that isn't required. You can do many at-home workouts if you don't want to join a gym. Just ensure you have the equipment and space to do it comfortably. On the same note, wear exercise-appropriate clothing. Find clothes that are comfortable and nonrestrictive. If you're doing impact-heavy exercises, ensure you have the right shoes to support your feet and legs to avoid injury.

Once you have the plan and have started putting it into action, sleep will follow as a natural consequence.

6

KEEP A SLEEP DIARY

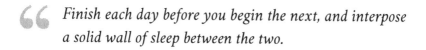 *Finish each day before you begin the next, and interpose a solid wall of sleep between the two.*

— RALPH WALDO EMERSON

WHAT IS A SLEEP DIARY?

Sleep diaries or journals are places we track and record sleep patterns and habits. They're largely used to measure sleep disorders, track symptoms, and identify patterns in your behavior. Sleep journals are kept over a specific period of time, usually several weeks. Doctors can use them to get an unbiased view of your sleeping habits. They can also be helpful for you to identify specific causes, find patterns in your behavior, and track progress with new treatments. It can be written on paper, typed into a document, or even logged into an app on your phone.

Think of your sleep diary as a place to collect clues to a mystery. Like a detective, you can use the information you collect in it to solve the mystery of your sleep issues.

BENEFITS OF A SLEEP DIARY

Firstly, a sleep journal is one of the best ways to diagnose sleep disorders accurately. Without it, doctors are limited by what a patient tells them. The issue is that most patients aren't looking for specific details that might differentiate one sleep disorder from another. As such, their descriptions of the problems can be vague and misleading. Again, doctors use sleep diaries to get a more detailed, unbiased view of your difficulties. The details contained in it can reveal important behavioral patterns and symptoms that might otherwise be overlooked. It also provides more context on important details. With all that information, a doctor can make better decisions and recommendations for your care.

Secondly, sleep journals track behavior and patterns that might be causing or contributing to your insomnia. These can be things that you aren't even aware of doing and thus never considered changing. Consistent tracking of your sleep behavior will help you identify what influences your sleep. It will give you insight into what you might be doing wrong and identify things you can change for better results.

Thirdly, journaling reduces stress. While a sleep diary can be used exclusively to track your patterns and symptoms, it can also double as a thought journal. We can do a lot with basic statistics and numbers, but they don't always illuminate what's happening in our heads. With that in mind, use your sleep diary to write out what makes you feel stressed and anxious. This way, you have an outlet for those thoughts, and you can see how those thoughts influence your sleep. If you're worried about sharing these with a doctor, don't be. Your mental state and stress impact your sleep, and this can be insightful knowledge for your doctor. For example, it could demonstrate that work stress is not the cause, but interpersonal tension is a strong contender.

Fourth, your sleep diary will monitor your progress and track the effectiveness of treatment strategies. The best way to know if something is working is to examine your progress objectively. There's a lot involved in managing sleep issues—it's not just a matter of feeling better. With a diary, you can see in detail how your sleep is changing, showing you whether a treatment strategy is working or not. This can help a lot in determining the best possible treatment plan. We don't have blood tests or X-rays to check our progress objectively, so instead, we use a sleep diary.

Lastly, sleep diaries are free and easy to use. They're also highly customizable. It's entirely up to you what to track and how to do it. You don't need anything special; the notes app on your phone or a separate notebook will do just fine.

THINGS TO WRITE IN A SLEEP DIARY

If you're keeping a diary at the request of a doctor or healthcare expert, they will likely tell you which details to include. If you're doing it on your own and without a premade template or app, make sure to note the following things:

- at what time you went to bed and when you tried to go to sleep
- how long it took to drift off
- how many times you woke up during the night
- how long, on average, it took you to fall back asleep at those times
- what time you wake up and when you get out of bed
- how many naps you took, if any, along with how long they lasted and at what times they occurred

Furthermore, you can rate how well you slept on a scale of one to ten, with ten meaning you woke up feeling well-rested

You should also track a few details about your day in your sleep diary. This will demonstrate how your daytime habits affect your sleep. Doing this can help you identify any factors that can cause or contribute to your insomnia, so keep note of these things. They might include

- how much caffeine, nicotine, and alcohol you had that day
- mealtimes, especially the last one of the day

- which medications you took (both prescription and over-the-counter) and how many you took. If possible, write down the dosage of that medication. For example, two Advil (ibuprofen 100mg each).
- energy levels throughout the day
- mood and stress
- how active you were throughout the day and whether you exercised
- what you did in the hours preceding your bedtime

Ideally, your sleep diary should be updated daily for consistent data. Try not to skip any days if you can help it. The more consecutive days you can track, the better. Don't fall into the trap of "I'll do it later."

DIARY DOS AND DON'TS

As helpful as a sleep journal can be, it can also cause stress and disruption. To ensure it is an aid and not a hindrance, let's review some tips for using your sleep diary.

- **Include both planned and unplanned daytime naps.** If you doze off by accident, it still counts as a nap, even if it was only for a few minutes. If you tried to nap but couldn't, write that down.
- **Track your sleep for at least two weeks before trying to interpret anything.** It takes time to get enough accurate information to start seeing patterns. Aim to get at least two weeks' worth of entries before reading through everything again. This is also true when you

use a diary to track new methods. These things need time to start working, so wait a while before trying to decide if it's working.

- **Leave your journal outside the bedroom before bed.** If it's close by, you might feel the urge to write in it every time you wake up during the night. It can even cause sleep latency simply by being nearby. Instead, leave it in the kitchen for some breakfast logging. The information doesn't have to be exact; you can write down approximations or your best guesses for things you can't remember with precision.

- **Fill daytime things in at the end of the day and sleep-related things the next morning.** Don't try to do a whole day's entry the next morning. By then, you may have forgotten something and thus might not get 100% accurate information.

- **Use fitness or sleep trackers if you have them.** Plenty of modern-day fitness trackers and smartwatches have built-in sleep monitors. Experiment with using them. They can often help give more accurate readings for things like wake times. Only wear them if they do not make you anxious about the information or are comfortable enough not to disturb your sleep. If you find yourself fiddling with them or wondering about them instead of sleeping, it's better to leave them off.

HOW TO INTERPRET A SLEEP DIARY

Sleep diaries are usually used over an extended period, such as weeks or months. While you are using it, make sure to note the same information every time. Find a template that works for you to ensure you list everything that's needed.

Every day, spend some time filling out the record. Start an entry with the date at the top, and then list all your necessary things. Keep repeating this for at least two weeks. Once that time has passed, look through the entries to find any patterns. Keep an eye out for

- how long you spend in bed compared to how long you sleep
- any habits that might influence your sleep behavior
- changes in your schedule that affect your sleep
- whether you are maintaining a regular schedule
- any common factors among days where you slept poorly
- any common characteristics among days you slept well that might be missing from bad days
- how your nighttime routine impacts your sleep. Is your sleep better or worse on days when you deviate from this routine?
- how your sleep compares to days you worked out versus days you didn't

Look for anything that might correlate to your sleep experience.

Use these results to find out what the optimum amount of sleep for you is, what routines have the best results, and which influences impact your sleep most. If you find any irregularities in your journal that you can't explain, bring them up with your doctor the next time you see them.

Once you have identified some possible influences, use them to make changes that will promote sleep. If you notice that you sleep worse on warm nights, for example, you can deduce that temperature influences your sleep and do something to manage it.

SLEEP DIARY TEMPLATES

If you're looking for a diary template, there are a few options to try. Finding a premade template online or using an app is easiest. If you're looking for inspiration, try searching *sleep diary templates* on Google and scrolling through the results.

There are two I recommend. The first is a two-week template from sleepeducation.org that has enough space to track 14 days (American Academy of Sleep Medicine, 2021). In this one, you record your activities at various times of the day.

The second is a daily template from the National Health Service (NHS) where you can fill in the answers to questions related to your sleep (Morgan, K. et al., 2007).

You can easily create your own if you don't want to use an existing template. Think beforehand about which details you want to track. In a word processor, create a table with enough rows for each question and enough columns for the days you want to track. Then, you can add the relevant information to it as you go. For example:

	Day 1	Day 2	Day 3	Day 4
What time did you go to bed?	10 p.m.			
How long did it take to fall asleep?	30 min			
How frequently did you wake up during the night?	3			

7

WHEN TO SEE A DOCTOR

> *Medical treatment is emergency care for symptoms that have developed over a long period of time. The symptom is the flower on a plant. Treating the symptom is picking the flower, while the plant remains untouched.*

— GARY ZUKAV

WHY IT'S IMPORTANT TO TREAT INSOMNIA

Sleep disorders might seem like a temporary inconvenience at first, but the longer they go unmanaged, the worse they will become. In other words, the longer insomnia goes untreated, the more damaging it becomes.

Untreated insomnia leads to sleep deprivation, and sleep deprivation leads to

- declining focus and concentration
- emotional instability
- worsening memory
- higher risk of accidents and injury
- a less fulfilling life

One research paper set out to list why insomnia needs to be treated as a condition and not just a symptom (Matteson-Rusby et al., 2010). The findings were as follows:

- Insomnia (especially chronic insomnia) does not resolve on its own.
- Chronic insomnia is debilitating. Referencing numerous other studies, this paper shows time and again how insomnia influences cognitive ability, social capacity, and vocational performance.
- Insomnia causes economic strain, both for individuals and society as a whole. Insomnia in the US is believed to cost more than $100 billion annually. Less than 15% of this is attributed to medical and pharmaceutical costs; the majority of this cost comes down to car and workplace accidents, absence from work, and lower job performance.
- Insomnia is common and affects a large percentage of people. It similarly affects a large portion of people, which in turn contributes to the economic cost of insomnia.

- Insomnia increases people's risk of developing physical and psychiatric health conditions. Overall, people who suffer from chronic insomnia are more likely to develop pain conditions, heart disease, high blood pressure, and gastrointestinal problems. This is believed to result in an increased mortality risk, though it remains untested. Other studies have found that chronic insomnia predisposes people to major depressive disorder.
- Insomnia treatments are generally safe, low-risk, and largely effective.

When you look at these factors, the question goes from "Why should I treat insomnia?" to "Why *not* treat insomnia?" It's a prevalent condition that affects millions of lives each year, with treatments that are as unharmful as they come. You have nothing to lose by seeking treatment.

WHEN TO SEE A SPECIALIST

A lot of the time, insomnia is something you can manage on your own without medical intervention. However, there are situations where it might be necessary to see a doctor about your sleep disruptions. This can be to get better help or access better care, or it can be because your symptoms are potentially dangerous. Insomnia isn't always a threatening condition; it's disruptive and debilitating, absolutely—but it isn't necessarily dangerous. Insomnia can be related to another serious condition, or it can lead to the development of serious, potentially dangerous consequences.

Seek medical attention if you relate to any of the following things:

- Your insomnia is chronic or lasts more than four weeks.
- Your symptoms interfere with your daily functioning.
- You experience symptoms of restless leg syndrome (i.e., a tingly or crawling feeling in your legs when you try to sleep.)
- You snore regularly or worry you might have sleep apnea.
- You notice excessive heartburn or feel physical pain that's keeping you awake.
- You experience excessive daytime sleepiness or fall asleep at unexpected times during the day.
- You feel distressed about your sleep issues.
- You see changes in your appetite, energy levels, and mood.
- You notice cataplexy (loss of control over muscles and movement) during the day.

Seek emergency medical care if you experience

- worsening physical pain
- difficulty breathing that wakes you up
- worsening mood to the point of suicidal or homicidal thoughts
- drifting off while performing dangerous tasks like driving or cooking

These scenarios indicate a more pressing issue and could indicate severe sleep deprivation.

WHAT TO EXPECT AT AN APPOINTMENT

If you see a doctor about sleep issues, they might refer you to a sleep clinic. Here, you will likely first go to an evaluation appointment. During this appointment, the specialist will ask you to answer a few questions, get your medical history, and perform a physical exam. These appointments aim to make the correct diagnosis and formulate the best possible treatment plan.

You might be asked to bring your bed partner along. A partner will be better able to answer questions about snoring, sleep-walking, or other nighttime behaviors.

Depending on the outcomes of the appointment, you might be recommended to have a sleep study performed. A sleep study is where you sleep in a controlled environment so doctors can monitor you while you are asleep. This helps them better understand the problem and allows them to monitor specific symptoms or vitals to prove or eliminate a diagnosis. During this study, sensors are attached to your skin to gauge vital signs like brain waves, heartbeat, and breathing.

You might also be asked to keep a sleep diary, wear a monitoring device at home, or make specific changes. Don't hesitate to ask if you're unsure about an appointment, test, or diagnosis.

Questions Your Doctor Might Ask

- How frequently do you experience sleep disturbances?
- How long has this persisted?
- At what time do you go to bed and wake up on workdays and on weekends?
- Do you wake up feeling tired or refreshed?
- How long does it take you to fall asleep at first and when you wake up during the night?
- Do you often drift off when you don't intend to sleep during the day?
- Has anyone told you that you snore or breathe weirdly during your sleep?
- Do you have any current or past health conditions, injuries, or incidents that might affect your sleep?
- What medications do you take?
- Do you consume caffeine, drink alcohol, or smoke?
- Do you exercise?
- How often do you travel long distances or experience jet lag?
- Are you experiencing stress?
- Do you have family members with sleep issues or disorders?
- Do you work irregular hours or night shifts?
- Are you feeling distressed about lack of sleep?
- What does your typical nighttime routine look like, and what do your dinners usually consist of?
- What does your sleep environment look like?

GET THE MOST OUT OF AN APPOINTMENT

Seeing a doctor is nerve-racking, even if you don't think anything bad is going to happen. Often, we go in looking for answers and then feel frustrated when we don't get what we expect. With that in mind, here are some tips to get the most out of the experience:

1. Be honest. Your doctor isn't going to judge you, so be open about your habits. Don't downplay your experiences or minimize your symptoms. Answer all questions truthfully to the best of your ability. Don't beat around the bush, omit things because you think it's irrelevant, or try to minimize things you think they might disapprove of. They aren't asking these things to shame you; they're asking because it's relevant to the diagnosis or treatment.

2. Bring someone with you, if you can. A second set of ears for a doctor's appointment is a great help. They can help you remember what was said, take notes, or offer moral support.

3. Write down your concerns or questions beforehand. A lot goes on in a doctor's appointment. If you have specific things you want to know or bring up, write them down before the appointment. This will help make sure everything necessary is addressed. Appointments are limited to a specific time, so it's best to have the things you want to prioritize clearly defined.

4. Ask for second opinions. Doctors are people, and as such, a second set of eyes is never a bad thing. Don't hesitate to ask for another opinion. Most doctors won't be offended by it. Getting a second opinion does not mean refusing or questioning their judgment; it simply means getting more insight into a problem and exploring all possible avenues.

5. Ask your questions and clarify information. If there's something you don't understand or something you want to ask, it is entirely within your rights to ask for clarification. Speak up if a doctor uses complex jargon or says something you don't understand. You can also repeat information back to them so they can confirm whether you understood it correctly. Don't worry about sounding stupid or being a bother; this is your life, and it's vital that you understand all information given to you. On the same note, don't be afraid to do some independent research. Ask your doctor to write down things like the diagnosis, treatment options, or medications, and then read up on those things on your own time.

TREATMENTS

Once a diagnosis has been made, your doctor will recommend a suitable treatment. The most common recommendation is to make the lifestyle changes discussed in previous chapters. Beyond that, there are other options as well.

Cognitive Behavioral Therapy (CBT)

CBT is a popular form of therapy that focuses on changing unhealthy and unrealistic beliefs and thought patterns. In the context of insomnia, CBT can be used to teach a person how to deal with the anxieties and feelings that might contribute to their insomnia.

This is a multifaceted therapy that can be used for many things. Depending on the context, symptoms, and patient, a trained therapist will use various strategies and methods to provide the best possible care. For insomnia, these tools can include the following:

- **Psychoeducation:** This is often the first tool used in most forms of CBT. Here, a patient learns all about sleep, their sleep patterns, and proper sleep hygiene. This is a learning stage where a patient and therapist can work together to establish a relationship and get on the same page.
- **Stimulus control:** This strategy aims to break the association between insomnia and your anxiety surrounding sleep. It seeks to make falling asleep easier by managing the stimulus that disrupts it. In this strategy, you'll be encouraged to stay out of bed unless you are sleeping, avoid naps, and get up if you can't sleep.
- **Sleep restriction and compression:** This technique aims to minimize the time a person spends in bed while awake.

- **Relaxation:** Here, a therapist will teach you effective relaxation exercises to help you unwind. I mentioned some of these exercises in Chapter 3.

Altogether, CBT is the standard treatment for insomnia. It teaches you how to make your mind work for you instead of against you. It is generally considered the best treatment option and is likely the one you'll be recommended first.

The reason it's so popular is that it is non-invasive, effective, and relatively low-risk. It doesn't just fix your sleep; it teaches you new coping mechanisms to manage the things that cause disruptions to your sleep.

Prescription or OTC Sleep Aids

As mentioned previously, sleeping pills can be beneficial in some cases. However, they are short-term solutions and will likely only be prescribed as a temporary measure. Your doctor might recommend taking some to help reset your sleep schedule. This can help break negative associations or implement healthier habits.

However, they are not intended to be a permanent solution and should not be your only form of treatment. Talk to your doctor about sleeping pills. Ensure you are informed of all the risks and benefits of the specific medication you take.

Lastly, use them as prescribed or instructed. Do not take more than the recommended dose or take them for longer periods than your doctor intended. If none are prescribed, talk to a doctor before taking any OTC sleep aid, especially if you take any other medication.

Integrative Medicine and Supplements

Integrative medicine refers to any other treatment, medication, or therapy that can work alongside other methods to manage insomnia. There are a lot of alternative treatment options for insomnia. Talk to your doctor about including them in your treatment plan if you want to.

- **Biofeedback therapy:** This is a kind of therapy where a practitioner tracks certain biological signals to look for a specific response. Patients can then learn to use those responses to affect changes in their bodies. It's believed that this can help you lower your heart rate, reduce blood pressure, steady breathing, and reduce muscle tension. These responses can thus be useful for falling asleep.

- **Herbal remedies:** Herbal supplements can improve your sleep. Some, like chamomile, have a proven sedative effect. Several herbal remedies are believed to reduce insomnia symptoms, including chamomile, valerian, kava, and passionflower. However, these supplements are not as well studied or controlled as pharmaceuticals and come with some risks. If you want to try an herbal supplement, talk to your doctor about it. They don't work equally in all circumstances, and knowing how these herbs will affect other medications or conditions is essential before experimenting with them.

- **Hypnosis:** Hypnosis is a form of therapy that uses the power of suggestion to affect changes in a person's behavior and to help them relax. Its use for insomnia is not well studied, but some research has shown that it can be helpful.
- **Massage:** A good massage can help you relax, but that isn't all there is to it. Look into different massage techniques to find ones that might help with your stress, health issues, and sleep disruptions. Research has shown that massage can be an effective tool for managing insomnia.
- **Acupuncture:** Acupuncture is a form of traditional medicine that uses needles to stimulate specific nerve points across the body. While it is not well-researched, it has been found to positively influence sleep.

HOW GREAT LIFE WOULD BE IF WE ALL HAD GOOD REST!

As you embrace healthy sleep habits, prioritize your fitness routine, and harness the benefits of a sleep diary, you will probably be keen to share the secrets of optimal sleep quality with others.

Simply by sharing your honest opinion of this book and a little about how its strategies helped you, you'll show new readers exactly where they can find the guidance they need to wake up in the morning filled with energy and a positive frame of mind.

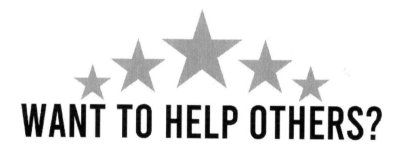

WANT TO HELP OTHERS?

Thank you so much for your support. Sleep is a solo effort – but sharing key strategies to boost sleep quantity and quality is something we can all do to help others lead healthier and happier lives.

CONCLUSION

Insomnia is tough—there's no way around it. It robs us of something elemental and important. It can cause damage in the long run, and many don't take it seriously enough. But it doesn't have to be this way. There are ways to manage it.

In this book, we covered a lot. We explored the mechanics of sleep, what insomnia is, and how our lifestyle influences it. Most importantly, we explored what we can do about it. So, what do you do now? **Start slowly and work your way into changing your habits**. It's a lot, I know. The best advice I can give you is to pick a place and start there. Change things one at a time. Start with something more manageable, then work up to the more difficult interventions.

You have taken the first steps along that journey. You opened yourself up to the possibility of treatment and sought out ways to get more information, and that's commendable. Armed with this knowledge, you can say goodbye to restless nights and tired days. All that's left to do is put it into action. Use what you've learned to carve out a better future.

Throughout it all, remember this: **You are not alone.** Millions of other people are experiencing the same struggle. Millions of others understand where you're at and know what you're going through. Millions of others have been and will be where you are now. They will get through this. Because you, too, can get through it.

If you found this book helpful, please consider leaving a review. Sharing your thoughts and experiences with me will help me improve future books. My goal with this book is to make information about insomnia and its treatments more accessible to those who might not have access to formal medical care.

My ultimate hope for you is to recover from this. I hope tossing and turning becomes a thing of the past. I hope the exhaustion and anxiety of sleeplessness become a distant memory. Most of all, I wish you a solid 7–9 hours of uninterrupted, blissful sleep.

REFERENCES

Acosta Scott, J. (2014, March 24). *The risks of taking sleeping pills.* EverydayHealth.com. https://www.everydayhealth.com/news/risks-taking-sleeping-pills/

Adopt good sleep habits. (2008, December 12). Division of Sleep Medicine at Harvard Medical School. https://healthysleep.med.harvard.edu/need-sleep/what-can-you-do/good-sleep-habits

American Academy of Sleep Medicine. (2021). *Two week sleep diary.* [Template]. Sleepeducation.org. https://sleepeducation.org/wp-content/uploads/2021/04/sleep-diary-form.pdf

American Psychological Association. (2023, March 8). *Stress effects on the body.* American Psychological Association. https://www.apa.org/topics/stress/body

Ask Apollo. (2022, October 10). *Stress - types, symptoms, causes, effects, prevention & management.* Apollo Hospitals Blog. https://healthlibrary.askapollo.com/stress-types-symptoms-causes-effects-management/

Asp, K. (2021, December 2). *How to quiet your mind to get better sleep.* EverydayHealth.com. https://www.everydayhealth.com/sleep/how-put-racing-mind-bed-sleep-now/

Avoiding those distractions at bedtime. (2022, October 18). Alaska Sleep Clinic. https://www.alaskasleep.com/~alaskasl/avoiding-those-distractions-at-bedtime-2/

AZ Quotes. (n.d.). Michael Xavier quotes. https://www.azquotes.com/quote/1088845

Baskin, K. (2017, October 27). *How to break the sleep-stress cycle.* MeQuilibrium. https://www.mequilibrium.com/resources/how-to-break-the-sleep-stress-cycle/

Bigley, J. (2021, December 3). *Sleep: How much you need and its 4 stages.* Cleveland Clinic. https://health.clevelandclinic.org/your-complete-guide-to-sleep/

Breus, D. M. (2023a, March 10). *The benefits of exercise for sleep.* The Sleep Doctor. https://thesleepdoctor.com/exercise/benefits-of-exercise-for-sleep/

Breus, D. M. (2023b, April 26). *Exercise at this time of day for optimal sleep*. The Sleep Doctor. https://thesleepdoctor.com/exercise/best-time-of-day-to-exercise-for-sleep/

Breus, M. (2022a, December 13). *How does alcohol affect sleep?* The Sleep Doctor. https://thesleepdoctor.com/alcohol-and-sleep/

Breus, M. (2022b, December 13). *The relationship between sleep and stress*. The Sleep Doctor. https://thesleepdoctor.com/mental-health/stress-and-sleep/

Breus, M. (2022c, December 13). *Why a regular sleep schedule matters to your health*. The Sleep Doctor. https://thesleepdoctor.com/sleep-hygiene/sleeping-schedule/

Breus, M. (2023, January 13). *What happens during sleep*. The Sleep Doctor. https://thesleepdoctor.com/sleep-faqs/what-happens-when-you-sleep/

Britton, A., Fat, L. N., & Neligan, A. (2020). The association between alcohol consumption and sleep disorders among older people in the general population. *Scientific Reports*, 10(1). https://doi.org/10.1038/s41598-020-62227-0

Brown, J. (2017, May 10). *8 sleep experts on what to do when you can't turn off your thoughts at night*. The Cut; The Cut. https://www.thecut.com/2017/05/8-sleep-experts-on-what-to-do-when-your-mind-is-racing.html

Buick, J. (2022, June 3). *Breaking the stress-sleep cycle*. Www.bupa.com.au. https://www.bupa.com.au/healthlink/mental-health-wellbeing/sleep/breaking-the-stress-sleep-cycle

Can just one drink ruin sleep? (2021, April 1). Sleep Dunwoody Blog. https://www.sleepdunwoody.com/blog/2021/04/01/can-just-one-drink-ruin-your-sleep/

Capritto, A. (2023, May 10). *4 workouts to help you sleep better tonight*. CNET. https://www.cnet.com/health/sleep/4-workouts-to-help-you-sleep-better/

Carlin, G. (1998). *Brain droppings*. Hyperion. (Original work published 1997)

Casper Editorial Team. (2019, December 19). *How to fix your sleep schedule: 14 data-backed tips*. Casper Blog. https://casper.com/blog/fix-sleep-schedule/

CDC. (2022, September 14). *How much sleep do I need? - Sleep and sleep disorders*. CDC; CDC. https://www.cdc.gov/sleep/about_sleep/how_much_sleep.html

Cherney, K. (2020, March 23). *Sleep disorder signs: When to see a specialist*.

Healthline. https://www.healthline.com/health/narcolepsy/see-a-sleep-specialist

Cherry, K. (2022, September 20). *Why cultivating a growth mindset can boost your success.* Verywell Mind. https://www.verywellmind.com/what-is-a-mindset-2795025

Chiam, J. (2023, March 8). *10 simple hacks to reducing alcohol intake for a better night's sleep.* Sunnyside. https://www.sunnyside.co/blog/sleep-hacks

Clear, J. (2013, June 24). *Fixed mindset vs growth mindset: How your beliefs change your behavior.* Jamesclear.com; James Clear. https://jamesclear.com/fixed-mindset-vs-growth-mindset

Cleveland Clinic. (2020, December 7). *Sleep basics: Rem, sleep stages, & more.* Cleveland Clinic. https://my.clevelandclinic.org/health/articles/12148-sleep-basics

Coelho, S. (2020, November 30). *Sleep cycle stages: Chart, durations, and how to improve sleep.* Www.medicalnewstoday.com. https://www.medicalnewstoday.com/articles/sleep-cycle-stages

Coelho, S. (2021, October 15). *A sleep diary could be the key to better rest.* Healthline. https://www.healthline.com/health/sleep/sleep-diary#what-are-they

Colrain, I. M., Nicholas, C. L., & Baker, F. C. (2014). Alcohol and the sleeping brain. *Handbook of Clinical Neurology, 125,* 415–431. https://doi.org/10.1016/b978-0-444-62619-6.00024-0

Corliss, J. (2022, February 2). *Six relaxation techniques to reduce stress.* Harvard Health. https://www.health.harvard.edu/mind-and-mood/six-relaxation-techniques-to-reduce-stress

Creveling, M. (2023, March 22). *How important is sticking to a sleep schedule, really?* Sleep.com. https://www.sleep.com/sleep-health/sleep-schedule

Crosta, P. (2023, January 9). *Insomnia: Causes, symptoms, and treatments.* Www.medicalnewstoday.com. https://www.medicalnewstoday.com/articles/9155

Cullins, A. (2022, July 9). *Fixed mindset vs. growth mindset examples.* Big Life Journal. https://biglifejournal.com/blogs/blog/fixed-mindset-vs-growth-mindset-examples

DeBara, D. (2022, March 28). *This simple mindset shift may help you get a better night's rest.* Fitbit Blog. https://blog.fitbit.com/mindset-shift-better-sleep/

Delgado, C. (2022, September 7). *Irregular sleep schedules can lead to health risks.*

Discover Magazine. https://www.discovermagazine.com/health/irregular-sleep-schedules-can-lead-to-health-risks

Deshong, A. (2022, December 13). *Sleep disorders.* The Sleep Doctor. https://thesleepdoctor.com/sleep-disorders/

Diaz, N., & Rohmiller , C. (n.d.). *How mindset impacts your education.* In Redefining Success. https://boisestate.pressbooks.pub/acad/chapter/how-mindset-impacts-your-education/

DiGiulio, S. (2017, October 19). *How what you eat affects your sleep.* NBC News; NBC News. https://www.nbcnews.com/better/health/how-what-you-eat-affects-how-you-sleep-ncna805256

DocDoc. (n.d.). *What is a sleep medicine consultation: Overview, benefits, and expected results.* DocDoc. https://www.docdoc.com/medical-information/procedures/sleep-medicine-consultation

Don't be shy: 4 tips for talking to your doctor. (n.d.). Www.hopkinsmedicine.org. https://www.hopkinsmedicine.org/health/wellness-and-prevention/dont-be-shy-4-tips-for-talking-to-your-doctor

Don't let perfectionism stop you from falling asleep easily. (2022, February 25). Www.beatrixaschmidt.com. https://www.beatrixaschmidt.com/blog/don-t-let-perfectionism-stop-you-from-falling-asleep-easily-treating-chronic-insomnia

Drillinger, M. (2020, March 3). *Why irregular sleep patterns may affect your heart health.* Healthline. https://www.healthline.com/health-news/irregular-sleep-patterns-increase-risk-of-heart-attack#Sleep-and-inflammation

Dunderman, G. (2023, March 23). *4 reasons to keep a sleep journal.* Clarity Clinic. https://www.claritychi.com/4-reasons-to-keep-a-sleep-journal/

Dusang, K. (2019, May 9). *How stress can affect your sleep.* Baylor College of Medicine. https://www.bcm.edu/news/how-stress-can-affect-your-sleep

The Editors of Encyclopaedia Britannica. (2001). Cytokine | biochemistry | Britannica. In *Encyclopædia Britannica.* https://www.britannica.com/science/cytokine

Elliott, B. (2020, August 27). *9 foods and drinks to promote better sleep.* Healthline. https://www.healthline.com/nutrition/9-foods-to-help-you-sleep

Erdman, S. (2013, August 22). *Relaxation techniques: Learn how to manage stress.* WebMD; WebMD. https://www.webmd.com/balance/guide/blissing-out-10-relaxation-techniques-reduce-stress-spot

Espie C., et al. (2014). *Insomnia questionnaire - sleep condition indicator (SCI).*

Www.sleepprimarycareresources.org.au. https://www.sleepprimarycarere sources.org.au/questionnaires/sci

EU Business School. (2022, June 2). *What's the difference between a growth mindset and a fixed mindset?* Euruni.edu. https://www.euruni.edu/blog/ whats-the-difference-between-a-growth-mindset-and-a-fixed-mindset/

Exercise programs. (2022, July 11). Vic.gov.au. https://www.betterhealth.vic. gov.au/health/HealthyLiving/exercise-programs

Familydoctor.org Editorial Staff. (2023, March 10). *Getting the most out of your doctor appointment.* Familydoctor.org. https://familydoctor.org/tips-for- talking-to-your-doctor/

Felman, A. (2020, October 1). *To snack or not to snack: What happens when you go to bed hungry.* Greatist. https://greatist.com/health/it-bad-sleep-empty- stomach#weight-loss

Fiverr. (2023, April 18). *When to seek medical care for insomnia.* MyDoc Urgent Care. https://mydocurgentcare.com/blog/when-to-seek-medical-care- for-insomnia/

Fogoros, R. N. (2023, March 15). *The role of the vagus nerve in the nervous system.* Verywell Health. https://www.verywellhealth.com/vagus-nerve- anatomy-1746123

France de Bravo, B., & Mohseni, K. (2018, October 15). *Can sleeping pills cause cancer?* National Center for Health Research. https://www.center4re search.org/trouble-sleeping-pills-not-safe-solution/

Francia, B. (2014, September 4). *Small daily improvements are key to long-term results.* Benfrancia.com. https://www.benfrancia.com/entrepreneurship- and-motivation/small-daily-improvements-key-long-term-results/

Freshwater, S. (2020, January 18). *3 types of stress and health hazards.* Shawna Freshwater, PhD. https://spacioustherapy.com/3-types-stress-health- hazards/

Friedman, W. (2023, January 12). *Types of stress and their symptoms - dealing with stress and anxiety management.* Mentalhelp.net. https://www.mental help.net/blogs/types-of-stress-and-their-symptoms/

Fulghum Bruce, D. (2008, July 13). *Understanding the side effects of sleeping pills.* WebMD. https://www.webmd.com/sleep-disorders/understanding-the- side-effects-of-sleeping-pills

Galbiati, A., Giora, E., Sarasso, S., Zucconi, M., & Ferini-Strambi, L. (2018). Repetitive thought is associated with both subjectively and objectively recorded polysomnographic indices of disrupted sleep in insomnia disorder. *Sleep Medicine, 45*, 55–61. https://doi.org/10.1016/j.sleep.2017.10.002

Get enough sleep. (2022, July 15). Health.gov; Office of Disease Prevention and Health Promotion. https://health.gov/myhealthfinder/healthy-living/mental-health-and-relationships/get-enough-sleep

Gilpin, R. (2023, May 11). *Going to bed hungry - is it A good or bad thing?* Sleep Advisor. https://www.sleepadvisor.org/going-to-bed-hungry/

Gravitate. (2018, April 15). *The benefits of a fitness program.* Totalhealthandfitness.com. https://www.totalhealthandfitness.com/the-benefits-of-a-fitness-program/

Hallal, F. (2021, July 6). *What time should you stop eating at night?* Healthline. https://www.healthline.com/nutrition/what-time-should-you-stop-eating#effects-of-eating-late

Happy. (2022, July 24). *Delta waves: What they are and why they're important.* Psychcrumbs.com. https://psychcrumbs.com/what-are-delta-waves/

He and She Eat Clean. (2019, August 26). *5 reasons why you need a fitness plan.* https://www.heandsheeatclean.com/5-reasons-why-you-need-a-fitness-plan

Healthline Editorial Team. (2020, February 25). *The basics of stress.* Healthline. https://www.healthline.com/health/stress

Holloway, C. (2020, November 11). *How exercise affects your sleep.* Health Essentials from Cleveland Clinic. https://health.clevelandclinic.org/how-exercise-affects-your-sleep/

How sleep works - how much sleep is enough? (2022, March 24). Www.nhlbi.nih.gov. https://www.nhlbi.nih.gov/health/sleep/how-much-sleep

How sleep works - why is sleep important? (2022, March 24). Www.nhlbi.nih.gov. https://www.nhlbi.nih.gov/health/sleep/why-sleep-important

How to break the cycle of stress and bad sleep. (n.d.). Www.otip.com. https://www.otip.com/Why-OTIP/News/How-to-break-the-cycle-of-stress-and-bad-sleep

Huang, T., Mariani, S., & Redline, S. (2020). Sleep irregularity and risk of cardiovascular events: The multi-ethnic study of atherosclerosis. *Journal of the American College of Cardiology, 75*(9), 991–999. https://doi.org/10.1016/j.jacc.2019.12.054

Hudson Therapy. (2020, November 9). *How to accept (and embrace) imperfection.*

Hudson Therapy Group. https://hudsontherapygroup.com/blog/how-to-accept-and-embrace-imperfection

Ingrassi, M. (2022, March 1). *How your bedroom design can affect your sleep.* Moretti Interior Design. https://morettiinteriordesign.com/blog/bedroom-interior-design/how-your-bedroom-design-can-affect-your-sleep/

Insomnia. (2022, February 13). Cleveland Clinic. https://my.clevelandclinic.org/health/diseases/12119-insomnia

Irregular sleep schedules can lead to bigger health issues. (2019, August 20). NIH MedlinePlus Magazine. https://magazine.medlineplus.gov/article/irregular-sleep-schedules-can-lead-to-bigger-health-issues

Jensen, D. (2021, April 22). *When should I exercise for the best sleep?* Sound Sleep Medical. https://www.soundsleepmedical.com/blog/when-should-i-exercise-for-the-best-sleep/

Johns Hopkins Medicine. (n.d.). *Exercising for better sleep.* Johns Hopkins Medicine. https://www.hopkinsmedicine.org/health/wellness-and-prevention/exercising-for-better-sleep

Johnson, J. (2018, September 5). *Stress and sleep: What's the link?* Www.medicalnewstoday.com. https://www.medicalnewstoday.com/articles/322994

Juergens, J. (2023, April 17). *Sleeping pill withdrawal and detox.* Addiction Center. https://www.addictioncenter.com/sleeping-pills/withdrawal-detox/

Kahn, J. (2022a, October 10). *What time should you stop eating before bed?* Www.risescience.com. https://www.risescience.com/blog/what-time-should-you-stop-eating-before-bed

Kahn, J. (2022b, December 22). *How long before bed should you stop drinking alcohol? Early.* Www.risescience.com. https://www.risescience.com/blog/how-long-before-bed-should-you-stop-drinking-alcohol

Karaev, P. (2022, September 19). *10 good foods to eat before bed for health and fitness.* Www.boxrox.com. https://www.boxrox.com/10-good-foods-to-eat-before-bed-for-health/

Kendall, B. (2020, March 7). *The role of perfectionism in chronic insomnia.* Www.bethkendall.com. https://www.bethkendall.com/blog/the-role-of-perfectionism-in-chronic-insomnia

Koller, T. (2017, March 17). *3 mindset changes that radically improved my sleep.* Thrive Global. https://medium.com/thrive-global/3-mindset-changes-

that-radically-improved-my-sleep-and-cured-my-insomnia-
466ba7c1944d

Kredlow, M. A., Capozzoli, M. C., Hearon, B. A., Calkins, A. W., & Otto, M.
W. (2015). The effects of physical activity on sleep: a meta-analytic review.
Journal of Behavioral Medicine, 38(3), 427–449. https://doi.org/10.1007/
s10865-015-9617-6

Kripke, D. F., Langer, R. D., & Kline, L. E. (2012). Hypnotics' association with
mortality or cancer: a matched cohort study. *BMJ Open, 2*(1). https://doi.
org/10.1136/bmjopen-2012-000850

Kubala, J. (2021, July 7). *6 foods that keep you awake at night.* Healthline. https://
www.healthline.com/nutrition/foods-that-keep-you-awake

Lauricella, C. J. (2022, July 28). *Exercise and sleep: Timing is everything.* https://
www.premierhealth.com/your-health/articles/women-wisdom-wellness-
/exercise-and-sleep-timing-is-everything

Lawler, M. (2022, September 16). *When you can't sleep: How to treat insomnia.*
EverydayHealth.com. https://www.everydayhealth.com/insomnia/what-
when-you-cant-sleep-all-about-insomnia-treatments/

Leech, J. (2023, April 25). *10 reasons why good sleep is important.* Healthline. https://
www.healthline.com/nutrition/10-reasons-why-good-sleep-is-important

Levi, R. (2022, December 13). *The benefits of keeping a sleep diary.* The Sleep
Doctor. https://thesleepdoctor.com/sleep-hygiene/sleep-diary/

Levitt, S. (2022, March 31). *How a sleep diary can help you uncover the secret to
better sleep.* Sleep.com. https://www.sleep.com/sleep-health/sleep-diary

Lim, M. (2017, October 19). *Learn how to sleep better by understanding sleep
cycles & stages.* Heveya® Singapore. https://www.heveya.sg/blogs/articles/
103744774-learn-how-to-sleep-better-by-understanding-sleep-cycles-
stages

Lin, H. H., Tsai, P. S., Fang, S. Y., & Liu, J. F. (2011). Effect of kiwifruit
consumption on sleep quality in adults with sleep problems. *Asia Pacific
Journal of Clinical Nutrition, 20*(2), 169–174. https://pubmed.ncbi.nlm.nih.
gov/21669584/

Lovering, C. (2022, February 15). *Insomnia myths and facts.* Healthline. https://
www.healthline.com/health/insomnia/insomnia-myths-facts

Lusk, V. (2023, March 16). *7 tips for talking to your doctor.* GoodRx. https://
www.goodrx.com/healthcare-access/patient-advocacy/tips-for-talking-
to-doctor-about-cost

MacDonald, A. (2015, October 30). *Using the relaxation response to reduce stress.* Harvard Health Blog. https://www.health.harvard.edu/blog/using-the-relaxation-response-to-reduce-stress-20101110780

Martin, S. (2008). *The power of the relaxation response.* Https://Www.apa.org. https://www.apa.org/monitor/2008/10/relaxation

Matteson-Rusby, S. E., Pigeon, W. R., Gehrman, P., & Perlis, M. L. (2010). Why treat insomnia? *Primary Care Companion to the Journal of Clinical Psychiatry, 12*(1). https://doi.org/10.4088/pcc.08r00743bro

Mayo Clinic Staff. (2016, October 15). Insomnia - symptoms and causes. Mayo Clinic. https://www.mayoclinic.org/diseases-conditions/insomnia/symptoms-causes/syc-20355167

Mayo Clinic Staff. (2021, March 24). *Stress management.* Mayo Clinic; Mayo Clinic. https://www.mayoclinic.org/healthy-lifestyle/stress-management/in-depth/stress-symptoms/art-20050987

Mayo Clinic Staff. (2022, April 28). *Relaxation techniques: Try these steps to reduce stress.* Mayo Clinic. https://www.mayoclinic.org/healthy-lifestyle/stress-management/in-depth/relaxation-technique/art-20045368

McCallum, K. (2021, October 1). *Caffeine & sleep: How long does caffeine keep you awake?* Www.houstonmethodist.org. https://www.houstonmethodist.org/blog/articles/2021/oct/caffeine-sleep-how-long-does-caffeine-keep-you-awake/

Meadows, A. (2023, May 4). *Treatments for insomnia.* Sleepfoundation.org. https://www.sleepfoundation.org/insomnia/treatment

Migala, J. (2022, February 1). *5 exercises that will help you get better sleep.* FitOn - #1 Free Fitness App, Stop Paying for Home Workouts. https://fitonapp.com/fitness/exercises-for-better-sleep/

Mikhail, A. (2022, August 6). *5 foods and drinks to avoid to get better sleep tonight.* Fortune Well. https://fortune.com/well/2022/08/06/5-foods-and-drinks-to-avoid-to-get-better-sleep-tonight/

Millard, E. (2021, March 4). *Irregular sleep schedules may be as bad as too little sleep.* Verywell Mind. https://www.verywellmind.com/irregular-sleep-schedules-as-bad-as-too-little-sleep-5114516

Mitchell, M. (2013). *Dr. Herbert Benson's relaxation response.* Psychology Today. https://www.psychologytoday.com/us/blog/heart-and-soul-healing/201303/dr-herbert-benson-s-relaxation-response

Moawad, H. (2021, December 14). *Daytime negative thoughts have an impact on sleep.* Psychiatric Times. https://www.psychiatrictimes.com/view/daytime-negative-thoughts-have-an-impact-on-sleep

Moore, C. (2015, December 23). *6 tips for talking to your doctor.* Www.healthgrades.com. https://www.healthgrades.com/right-care/patient-advocate/6-tips-for-talking-to-your-doctor

Moore, P. (2022, March 23). *How to change your mindset about sleep.* WebMD. https://www.webmd.com/sleep-disorders/features/change-your-sleep-mindset

Morgan, K., David, B., & Gascoigne, C. (2007). *Daily sleep diary.* [Template]. Loughborough University Clinical Sleep Research Unit. https://www.nhs.uk/Livewell/insomnia/Documents/sleepdiary.pdf

Morrison, M. (2021, October 18). *6 tips for talking to your doctor.* Oak Street Health. https://www.oakstreethealth.com/6-tips-for-talking-to-your-doctor-624293

Morse, R. (n.d.). *The importance of sleep schedules.* Www.thejoint.com. https://www.thejoint.com/georgia/peachtree-corners/peachtree-corners-04047/306312-importance-sleep-schedules

Mulla, R. (2020, August 6). *How negative thinking can disrupt your sleep.* Www.sleepstation.org.uk. https://www.sleepstation.org.uk/articles/sleep-tips/self-fulfilling-prophecies/

Mulla, R. (2021, December 6). *Overthinking: Can't sleep? How thought blocking can help.* Www.sleepstation.org.uk. https://www.sleepstation.org.uk/articles/sleep-tips/thought-blocking/

Nagle, B. (2021, March 22). *What to expect at a consultation.* MultiCare. https://www.multicare.org/services-and-departments/sleep-medicine/how-we-help/what-to-expect-at-a-consultation/

National Institute of Neurological Disorders and Stroke. (2022, September 26). *Brain basics: Understanding sleep.* Www.ninds.nih.gov. https://www.ninds.nih.gov/health-information/public-education/brain-basics/brain-basics-understanding-sleep

National Institutes of Health . (2019, June 5). *Study links irregular sleep patterns to metabolic disorders.* Www.nih.gov. https://www.nih.gov/news-events/news-releases/study-links-irregular-sleep-patterns-metabolic-disorders

Navab, P. (2023, February 9). *How to stop catastrophic thinking at bedtime.* Time. https://time.com/6253219/how-to-stop-catastrophic-thinking-sleep/

NHLBI. (2019, June 5). *Irregular sleep patterns linked to higher risk of metabolic disorders.* Www.nhlbi.nih.gov. https://www.nhlbi.nih.gov/news/2019/

irregular-sleep-patterns-linked-higher-risk-metabolic-disorders

NHS self assessment. (n.d.). Assets.nhs.uk. https://assets.nhs.uk/tools/self-assessments/index.mob.html?variant=72

O'Keefe Osborn, C. (2018, July 31). *How to sober up (and 3 myths that won't help).* Healthline. https://www.healthline.com/health/how-to-sober-up#what-to-do-before-bed

Okoye, A. (2022, December 13). *Why a regular sleep schedule matters to your health.* The Sleep Doctor. https://thesleepdoctor.com/sleep-hygiene/sleeping-schedule/

Olson, E. J. (2023, February 21). *How many hours of sleep do you need?* Mayo Clinic. https://www.mayoclinic.org/healthy-lifestyle/adult-health/expert-answers/how-many-hours-of-sleep-are-enough/faq-20057898

Osmun, R. (2015, January 28). *5 ways to kick away negative thoughts before sleeping.* Lifehack. https://www.lifehack.org/articles/lifestyle/5-ways-kick-away-negative-thoughts-before-sleeping.html

Osmun, R. (2023, April 20). *9 ways to optimize your bedroom for better sleep.* Amerisleep.com. https://amerisleep.com/blog/optimize-bedroom-better-sleep/

Pacheco, D. (2020, September 4). *Alcohol and sleep.* Sleep Foundation. https://www.sleepfoundation.org/nutrition/alcohol-and-sleep

Pacheco, D. (2022, May 6). *The best aerobic exercises to get better sleep.* Sleep Foundation. https://www.sleepfoundation.org/physical-activity/best-exercises-sleep

Pacheco, D. (2023a, March 3). *The best time of day to exercise for sleep.* Sleep Foundation. https://www.sleepfoundation.org/physical-activity/best-time-of-day-to-exercise-for-sleep

Pacheco, D. (2023b, March 17). *Caffeine & sleep problems.* Sleep Foundation. https://www.sleepfoundation.org/nutrition/caffeine-and-sleep

Pacheco, D. (2023c, March 17). *Side effects of sleeping pills - Are they bad for you?* Sleep Foundation. https://www.sleepfoundation.org/sleep-aids/side-effects-of-sleeping-pills

Pacheco, D. (2023d, March 17). *What to snack on before bed.* Sleep Foundation. https://www.sleepfoundation.org/nutrition/healthy-bedtime-snacks

Pacheco, D. (2023e, March 24). *Exercise and sleep.* Sleep Foundation. https://www.sleepfoundation.org/physical-activity/exercise-and-sleep

Pacheco, D. (2023f, May 5). *Bedroom environment: What elements are important?* Sleep Foundation. https://www.sleepfoundation.org/bedroom-environment

Palahniuk, C. (2018). *Fight Club*. W.W. Norton & Company. (Original work published 1996)

Paprocki, J. (2018, January 29). *Sleep and caffeine*. Sleep Education. https://sleepeducation.org/sleep-caffeine/

Passos, G. S., Poyares, D. L., Santana, M. G., Tufik, S., & Mello, M. T. (2012). Is exercise an alternative treatment for chronic insomnia? *Clinics, 67*(6), 653–659. https://doi.org/10.6061/clinics/2012(06)17

Patrick, K. (2021, May 5). *3 mindset techniques to reclaim your sleep.* Entrepreneur. https://www.entrepreneur.com/living/3-mindset-techniques-to-reclaim-your-sleep/367820

Pediatric IBD Center. (2019, October 15). *Tips to manage stress with the relaxation response.* Massachusetts General Hospital. https://www.massgeneral.org/children/inflammatory-bowel-disease/tips-to-manage-stress-with-the-relaxation-response

Peters, B. (2021, September 10). *Consider 5 factors to create an optimal bedroom environment for sleep.* Verywell Health. https://www.verywellhealth.com/the-importance-of-your-sleep-environment-3014944

Peters, B. (2022, June 13). *Discover how to use a sleep log or sleep diary to diagnose insomnia.* Verywell Health. https://www.verywellhealth.com/sleep-log-sleep-disorder-diagnostic-tool-3015120

Peters, B. (2023a, January 18). *Is late coffee ruining your sleep?* Verywell Health. https://www.verywellhealth.com/how-long-should-you-wait-between-caffeine-and-bedtime-3014980

Peters, B. (2023b, May 13). *Timing of last meal may contribute to nighttime heartburn or insomnia.* Verywell Health. https://www.verywellhealth.com/eating-before-bed-3014981

Pritchard, K. (2020, October 27). *How exercise can help you sleep better.* Eachnight.com. https://eachnight.com/sleep/exercise-and-sleep/

Rally. (2017, July 25). *The importance of a sleep schedule.* SLMA. https://www.slma.cc/the-importance-of-a-sleep-schedule/

Ralph Waldo Emerson quotes. (n.d.). Quoteslyfe.com. https://www.quoteslyfe.com/quote/Finish-each-day-before-you-begin-the-982966

Ramakrishnan, K., & Scheid, D. C. (2007). Treatment options for insomnia. *American Family Physician, 76*(4), 517–526. https://www.aafp.org/pubs/afp/issues/2007/0815/p517.html

Rawls, B. (2022, February 24). *Stressed and sleepless? 11 unique ways to break the vicious cycle.* Vital Plan | The Power of Nature in Your Hands. https:// vitalplan.com/blog/stressed-and-sleepless-11-unique-ways-to-break-the-vicious-cycle

Ray, A. (2015). *Mindfulness : living in the moment, living in the breath.* Inner Light Publishers.

The Recovery Village. (2022a, May 26). *7 common myths about insomnia.* The Recovery Village Drug and Alcohol Rehab. https://www.therecoveryvil lage.com/mental-health/insomnia/insomnia-myths/

The Recovery Village. (2022b, May 26). *Insomnia facts & statistics.* The Recovery Village Drug and Alcohol Rehab. https://www.therecoveryvil lage.com/mental-health/insomnia/insomnia-statistics/

Reed, M. (2015, May 19). *How to eliminate negative sleep thoughts.* Healthcentral.com. https://www.healthcentral.com/article/how-to-elimi nate-negative-sleep-thoughts

Regan, S. (2022, May 6). *Want to stay asleep through the entire night? Avoid these 6 foods before bed.* Mindbodygreen. https://www.mindbodygreen.com/arti cles/foods-to-avoid-before-bed

Robb-Dover, K. (2022, June 18). *5 tips to quit using sleeping pills.* Fherehab.com. https://fherehab.com/learning/tips-quit-using-sleeping-pills

Rosenberg, C. (2019, July 17). *9 foods to avoid before bed.* Https://Www.sleep-healthsolutionsohio.com/. https://www.sleephealthsolutionsohio.com/ blog/foods-avoid-before-sleep/

Ruth. (2022, October 13). *How do I use a sleep diary with my child?* Support for Parents from Action for Children. https://parents.actionforchildren.org. uk/sleep/improving-sleep/sleep-diary-child/

Rutherford-Morrison, L. (2016, July 28). *6 unexpected things in your bedroom that affect the way you sleep.* Bustle. https://www.bustle.com/articles/ 174737-6-unexpected-things-in-your-bedroom-that-affect-the-way-you-sleep

Salter, O. (2023, April 6). *Does alcohol affect sleep quality?* Nature's Best. https:// www.naturesbest.co.uk/pharmacy/sleep-health/does-alcohol-affect-sleep-quality/

Say, J. (2022, November 16). *Top 39 sleep quotes to calm you.* Gracious Quotes. https://graciousquotes.com/sleep/

Scott, E. (2020, March 12). *Relaxation response for reversing stress.* Verywell Mind. https://www.verywellmind.com/what-is-the-relaxation-response-3145145

Scott, E. (2021, July 9). *How exactly does stress affect sleep?* Verywell Mind. https://www.verywellmind.com/relationship-between-stress-and-sleep-3144945

Scott, E. (2022, November 7). *What is stress?* Verywell Mind. https://www.verywellmind.com/stress-and-health-3145086

Scott, E. (2023, February 27). *10 telltale signs you may be a perfectionist.* Verywell Mind. https://www.verywellmind.com/signs-you-may-be-a-perfectionist-3145233

The science of sleep: Understanding what happens when you sleep. (n.d.). Johns Hopkins Medicine Health Library. https://www.hopkinsmedicine.org/health/wellness-and-prevention/the-science-of-sleep-understanding-what-happens-when-you-sleep

Sedative-hypnotic. (2007). *The American Heritage® Medical Dictionary.* https://medical-dictionary.thefreedictionary.com/sedative-hypnotic

Sen, S. (2023, March 13). *How exercise can help you sleep better.* Amerisleep.com. https://amerisleep.com/blog/exercise-and-sleep/

Sexton, A. (1971). *Transformations.* Houghton Mifflin Company.

Simpson , K. (2023, February 14). *How to fix your sleep schedule (circadian rhythm).* Sleep Advisor. https://www.sleepadvisor.org/how-to-fix-sleep-schedule/

Sleep and caffeine. (2022, November 23). Health Navigator New Zealand. https://www.healthnavigator.org.nz/healthy-living/s/sleep-and-caffeine/

SleepHealth. (2023, March 20). *The importance of sleep and understanding sleep stages.* Sleephealth.org. https://www.sleephealth.org/sleep-health/importance-of-sleep-understanding-sleep-stages/

Sleeping pills and how to safely stop. (2020, December 15). SaferMedsNL. https://safermedsnl.ca/sleeping-pills-how-to-safely-stop

SleepScore Labs. (2021, November 11). *The untold value of keeping a sleep diary.* SleepScore. https://www.sleepscore.com/blog/benefits-sleep-diary/

Slideshow: Insomnia myths and facts. (2022, June 26). WebMD. https://www.webmd.com/sleep-disorders/ss/slideshow-insomnia

Smith, J. (2020, September 25). *Growth vs fixed mindset: How what you think affects what you achieve.* Mindset Health. https://www.mindsethealth.com/matter/growth-vs-fixed-mindset

Spector, N. (2018, September 24). *How to beat back night-time anxiety and get some sleep.* NBC News. https://www.nbcnews.com/better/pop-culture/how-beat-back-night-time-anxiety-get-sleep-ncna912621

Stanwyck, M. (2020, July 30). *4 benefits of having a workout plan*. Whole Life Challenge. https://www.wholelifechallenge.com/4-benefits-of-having-workout-plan/

Stewart, K. (2022, March 2). *How to fix your sleep schedule*. EverydayHealth.com. https://www.everydayhealth.com/sleep/insomnia/resetting-your-clock.aspx

Stobo, R. (2022, January 27). *Snooze, don't lose: Here's how to fix your sleep schedule*. Greatist. https://greatist.com/health/how-to-fix-sleep-schedule

Strycharczyk, D. (2019, April 2). *How your mindset can affect your sleep*. AQR International. https://aqrinternational.co.uk/how-your-mindset-can-affect-your-sleep

Summer, J. (2022, April 15). *Eight health benefits of sleep*. Sleep Foundation; Jay Summer. https://www.sleepfoundation.org/how-sleep-works/benefits-of-sleep

Suni, E. (2020, November 6). *Nutrition and sleep: Diet's effect on sleep*. Sleep Foundation. https://www.sleepfoundation.org/nutrition

Suni, E. (2022a). *What causes insomnia?* Sleepfoundation.org. https://www.sleepfoundation.org/insomnia/what-causes-insomnia

Suni, E. (2022b, April 19). *Can overeating cause sleep disturbances?* Sleep Foundation. https://www.sleepfoundation.org/physical-health/sleep-and-overeating

Suni, E. (2022c, December 15). *Technology in the bedroom*. Sleep Foundation. https://www.sleepfoundation.org/bedroom-environment/technology-in-the-bedroom

Suni, E. (2023a, March 2). *Stages of sleep: What happens in a sleep cycle*. Sleep Foundation. https://www.sleepfoundation.org/stages-of-sleep

Suni, E. (2023b, March 3). *Insomnia*. Sleep Foundation. https://www.sleepfoundation.org/insomnia

Suni, E. (2023c, March 22). *How much sleep do we really need?* Sleep Foundation. https://www.sleepfoundation.org/how-sleep-works/how-much-sleep-do-we-really-need

Suni, E. (2023d, March 31). *How to reset your sleep routine: Tips & tricks*. Sleep Foundation. https://www.sleepfoundation.org/sleep-hygiene/how-to-reset-your-sleep-routine

Suni, E. (2023e, March 31). *What is sleep hygiene?* Sleep Foundation. https://www.sleepfoundation.org/sleep-hygiene

Suni, E. (2023f, April 25). *100+ sleep statistics - facts and data about sleep 2023*.

Sleep Foundation. https://www.sleepfoundation.org/how-sleep-works/sleep-facts-statistics#statistics-about-sleep-disorders-3

Sweeney, E. (2022, October 21). *Exercise really can help you sleep better at night – here's why that may be.* The Conversation. https://theconversation.com/exercise-really-can-help-you-sleep-better-at-night-heres-why-that-may-be-192427

TB. (2017, July 3). *Discover how mindsets influence our behavior.* Success, Financial Freedom & Building Wealth. https://topquestionsandanswers.com/home/2017/7/2/discover-how-mindsets-influence-our-behavior

Tiwari, D. (2023, April 4). *3 types of stress: Causes, effects, & how to cope.* Choosing Therapy. https://www.choosingtherapy.com/types-of-stress/

Toholka, K. (2016, May 22). *5 tips to accept your imperfections, no matter how different you feel.* Tiny Buddha. https://tinybuddha.com/blog/5-tips-accept-imperfections-no-matter-how-different-you-feel/

Tracy. (2023, April 8). *Are you too perfect to sleep? Perfectionism and insomnia.* Tracy the Sleep Coach. https://www.tracythesleepcoach.co.uk/are-you-too-perfect-to-sleep-perfectionism-and-insomnia/

True Personal Training. (2021, June 17). *The benefits of a workout plan.* Www.truepersonaltraining.co.uk. https://www.truepersonaltraining.co.uk/b/benefits-of-a-workout-plan

Understanding insomnia: Causes and Coping. (2022, May 25). Www.baptisthealth.com. https://www.baptisthealth.com/blog/family-health/understanding-insomnia-causes-and-coping

Vadlamani, S. (2021, March 19). *Embrace imperfection: Six ways to celebrate your flaws.* Happiness.com. https://www.happiness.com/magazine/personal-growth/embrace-your-imperfections/

Vogel, K. (n.d.). *Are these nighttime distractions ruining your sleep?* Happify.com. https://www.happify.com/hd/6-sleep-distractions-and-what-to-do-about-them/

Waters, S. (2022, August 25). *Types of stress and what you can do to fight them.* Www.betterup.com. https://www.betterup.com/blog/types-of-stress

Watson, S. (2021, July 12). *Keeping a sleep diary.* WebMD. https://www.webmd.com/sleep-disorders/how-to-use-a-sleep-diary#1

WebMD. (2006, December 31). *When to seek medical care for insomnia.* https://www.webmd.com/sleep-disorders/insomnia-when-to-go-to-doctor

WebMD. (2011, August 2). *Insomnia: Questions & answers for your doctor.*

https://www.webmd.com/sleep-disorders/insomnia-questions-for-doctor

WebMD. (2021, December 8). *The effects of stress on your body.* https://www.webmd.com/balance/stress-management/effects-of-stress-on-your-body

WebMD. (2022, September 8). *Exercises for better sleep.* https://www.webmd.com/sleep-disorders/ss/exercises-better-sleep

WebMD Editorial Contributors. (2011, February 9). *Understanding insomnia.* https://www.webmd.com/sleep-disorders/insomnia-overview

What are the effects of alcohol on sleep? (n.d.). Priory. https://www.priorygroup.com/blog/what-are-the-effects-of-alcohol-on-sleep

What to expect at your sleep study. (2021, February 11). Department of Neurology. https://www.med.unc.edu/neurology/divisions/sleep-1/frequently-asked-questions/what-to-expect-at-your-sleep-study/

When is the best time to exercise for great sleep? (2020, January 9). Healthily. https://www.livehealthily.com/sleep/when-is-the-best-time-to-exercise-for-great-sleep

Why it's so important to treat insomnia. (2021, January 27). Sleep Dunwoody Blog. https://www.sleepdunwoody.com/blog/2019/08/05/why-its-so-important-to-treat-insomnia/

Wiesel, E. (2006). *Night* (M. Wiesel, Trans.). Hill and Wang. (Original work published 1958)

Zhang, Y., Cordina-Duverger, E., Komarzynski, S., Attari, A. M., Huang, Q., Aristizabal, G., Faraut, B., Léger, D., Adam, R., Guénel, P., Brettschneider, J. A., Finkenstädt, B. F., & Lévi, F. (2022). Digital circadian and sleep health in individual hospital shift workers: A cross sectional telemonitoring study. *EBioMedicine,* 81(104121). https://doi.org/10.1016/j.ebiom.2022.104121

Zukav, G., & Francis, L. (2012). *Thoughts from the heart of the soul.* Simon and Schuster.

Zwarensteyn, J. (2022, October 3). *How do you get off sleeping pills? - symptoms & what to expect.* Sleep Advisor. https://www.sleepadvisor.org/how-to-get-off-sleeping-pills/

Printed in Great Britain
by Amazon

37292117R00093